WEIGHT LOSS FOR HOPELESS CASES

TURNING DESPAIR INTO TRIUMPH

INTRODUCTION

Introduction: Understanding the Challenge

1. The Struggles of Weight Loss

The Complexity of Weight Loss

Weight loss is not a simple matter of eating less and moving more. It's a complex interplay of various factors, including genetics, metabolism, hormones, behavior, and environment. For many, the journey is fraught with obstacles that can make the process seem daunting and, at times, impossible. Recognizing the multifaceted nature of weight loss is crucial for developing a comprehensive approach to overcoming these challenges.

Common Struggles

- **Emotional Eating:** Many individuals use food as a coping mechanism for stress, boredom, or emotional distress. This can lead to a cycle of overeating and guilt that is difficult to break.

- **Lack of Time:** Busy lifestyles can make it challenging to find time for meal planning, grocery shopping, and exercise. Convenience foods, which are often unhealthy, become the go-to option.
- **Inconsistent Motivation:** Motivation can wane over time, especially if results are not immediate. This inconsistency can lead to abandoned diets and exercise routines.
- **Plateaus:** Even with consistent effort, weight loss can sometimes stall, leading to frustration and a sense of failure.
- **Social Pressures:** Social gatherings and cultural norms can create environments where unhealthy eating is encouraged, making it difficult to stick to healthy choices.
- **Medical Conditions:** Certain medical conditions, such as thyroid disorders or polycystic ovary syndrome (PCOS), can make weight loss more challenging.

2. Why Some Feel Hopeless

Previous Failures

Repeated attempts to lose weight that end in failure can erode confidence and create a sense of hopelessness. Each failed attempt can reinforce the belief that losing weight is impossible, leading to a cycle of trying and giving up.

Unrealistic Expectations

Many people embark on weight loss journeys with unrealistic expectations, often fueled by media portrayals of rapid transformations and "quick-fix" solutions. When these expectations are not met, it can lead to discouragement and the belief that they are incapable of losing weight.

Negative Self-Image

A negative self-image can be both a cause and a result of weight issues. Individuals who have struggled with their weight for a long time may internalize negative beliefs about themselves, which can undermine their efforts and contribute to feelings of hopelessness.

Lack of Support

Support from family, friends, and the community can play a significant role in weight loss success. Without this support, individuals may feel isolated and overwhelmed by the challenges they face.

3. The Science of Weight Gain and Loss

Energy Balance

At its core, weight management is about energy balance—calories consumed versus calories expended. When you consume more calories than your body needs for maintenance and activity, the excess is stored as fat. Conversely, creating a calorie deficit by consuming fewer calories than you expend leads to weight loss.

Metabolism

Metabolism refers to all the chemical processes that occur within the body to maintain life, including converting food into energy. Basal metabolic rate (BMR) is the number of calories your body needs to perform basic functions at rest, such as breathing and maintaining body temperature. Factors influencing metabolism include age, sex, muscle mass, and genetics.

Hormones

Hormones play a crucial role in regulating appetite, metabolism, and fat storage. For instance:

- **Insulin:** Helps regulate blood sugar levels. Excess insulin can promote fat storage and hinder weight loss.
- **Leptin:** Signals satiety and helps regulate energy balance. Leptin resistance, common in obesity, can lead to overeating.
- **Ghrelin:** Known as the "hunger hormone," it stimulates appetite. Ghrelin levels increase before meals and decrease after eating.

Genetics

Genetics can influence various aspects of weight, including where you store fat, how your body processes food, and your appetite. While genetics can predispose individuals to weight gain, they do not make weight loss impossible. Understanding your genetic predispositions can help tailor your approach to weight loss.

4. Overview of the Book

Purpose

This book aims to provide a comprehensive guide to weight loss for those who feel hopeless. It acknowledges the unique challenges faced by individuals who have struggled with their weight for years, offering practical, science-based strategies to overcome these obstacles.

Structure

The book is divided into 20 chapters, each focusing on a different aspect of weight loss. Every chapter contains four subchapters that delve deeper into specific topics, providing detailed guidance and actionable steps.

1. **The Mindset Shift:** Addresses the psychological aspects of weight loss, including identifying limiting beliefs, cultivating positivity, practicing self-compassion, and setting realistic goals.
2. **Nutrition Basics:** Covers the fundamentals of nutrition, including understanding macronutrients and micronutrients, debunking diet myths, and creating a balanced meal plan.

3. **Emotional Eating:** Explores strategies to manage emotional eating, recognize triggers, develop healthy coping mechanisms, and build a support system.

4. **Exercise Essentials:** Provides guidance on finding the right exercise, incorporating movement into daily life, balancing strength training and cardio, and creating a sustainable routine.

5. **Breaking Through Plateaus:** Discusses how to identify and overcome weight loss plateaus by adjusting diet and exercise routines and staying motivated.

6. **Overcoming Medical and Genetic Challenges:** Examines the impact of medical conditions and genetics on weight loss and offers tailored strategies to address these challenges.

7. **Building Healthy Habits:** Focuses on the science of habit formation, making small changes for big results, creating a daily routine, and tracking progress.

8. **The Importance of Sleep:** Highlights the connection between sleep and weight, strategies for improving sleep quality, and managing sleep disorders.

9. **Stress Management:** Discusses how stress affects weight, techniques for stress reduction, and incorporating mindfulness and relaxation practices.

10. **Understanding Metabolism:** Explains metabolism, factors affecting it, ways to boost metabolic rate, and debunks common myths.

11. **Social Influences on Weight Loss:** Offers strategies for navigating social pressures, building a support network, dealing with sabotage, and celebrating successes.

12. **The Role of Technology:** Explores the use of apps and gadgets, online communities, and staying informed with the latest research.

13. **The Psychological Aspect:** Addresses body image, the role of therapy, developing a healthy relationship with food, and overcoming negative self-talk.

14. **Customizing Your Plan:** Guides you in assessing your needs, creating a personalized strategy, adapting as you progress, and maintaining flexibility.

15. **The Long-Term Perspective:** Prepares you for maintaining weight loss, preventing regain, continuing healthy habits, and setting new goals.

16. **Inspiring Success Stories:** Shares real-life transformations, common success strategies, and ways to stay inspired.

17. **The Role of Professional Help:** Discusses working with nutritionists, personal trainers, seeking psychological support, and using medical interventions wisely.

18. **Addressing Common Pitfalls:** Identifies potential roadblocks, strategies to overcome

them, staying consistent, and learning from setbacks.

19. **Celebrating Milestones:** Encourages recognizing non-scale victories, rewarding efforts, reflecting on your journey, and planning for the future.

20. **Embracing a New Lifestyle:** Focuses on making permanent changes, fostering a healthy environment, spreading positive influence, and continuing self-improvement.

Approach

This book takes a holistic approach to weight loss, addressing not just diet and exercise, but also the mental, emotional, and social factors that contribute to weight gain and loss. It combines scientific research with practical advice, offering a realistic and sustainable path to weight loss.

By understanding the multifaceted nature of weight loss and acknowledging the unique challenges faced by those who feel hopeless, this book aims to provide the tools, strategies, and support necessary to achieve lasting success. Each chapter builds on the foundation of the previous ones, creating a comprehensive and cohesive guide to transforming your body and mind.

1

THE MINDSET SHIFT

1. Identifying Limiting Beliefs

Understanding Limiting Beliefs

Many individuals embark on their weight loss journey with an array of preconceived notions and limiting beliefs that can severely hinder their progress. These beliefs are often deeply ingrained and can stem from various sources such as past experiences, societal influences, family dynamics, and internal dialogues. Examples of limiting beliefs might include:

- "I've always been overweight; it's just who I am."
- "I've tried dieting before, and it never works for me."
- "I don't have the willpower to stick to a diet."
- "Healthy eating is too expensive and complicated."

To identify these beliefs, it's essential to engage in self-reflection. Journaling can be a powerful tool in this process. Start by writing down your thoughts and feelings about weight loss and examine the language you use. Are there negative patterns or recurring themes? Recognizing these limiting beliefs is the first step in addressing and transforming them.

Challenging Limiting Beliefs

Once you have identified your limiting beliefs, the next step is to challenge them. This involves questioning the validity of these beliefs and considering alternative perspectives. Ask yourself:

- **Is this belief based on fact or assumption?** Often, limiting beliefs are not grounded in reality but are rather assumptions we've made based on past experiences or societal messages.
- **What evidence do I have that contradicts this belief?** Look for instances where you or others have successfully lost weight or made positive changes despite similar challenges.
- **How is this belief serving me?** Sometimes, limiting beliefs can serve as a protective mechanism, preventing us from taking risks or facing potential failure. Acknowledge this but also recognize that holding onto these beliefs can be more harmful in the long run.

Replacing limiting beliefs with empowering ones is crucial. For instance, if you believe "I don't have the willpower," reframe it to "I am capable of developing stronger willpower with practice and support."

Affirmations and Positive Self-Talk

Affirmations are positive statements that can help reinforce new, empowering beliefs. Create a list of affirmations that resonate with you and repeat them daily. Examples include:

- "I am committed to my health and well-being."
- "Every day, I am becoming stronger and healthier."
- "I have the power to make positive changes in my life."

Pair these affirmations with positive self-talk. When you catch yourself engaging in negative self-talk, consciously replace those thoughts with positive, encouraging ones. Over time, this practice can help shift your mindset and reinforce a more positive outlook.

2. Cultivating a Positive Attitude

The Role of Positivity in Weight Loss

A positive attitude is a critical component of any successful weight loss journey. It involves focusing on what you can achieve rather than what you can't, and it's about maintaining hope and motivation even in the face of challenges. Positivity helps reduce stress, improves resilience, and enhances overall well-being, all of which are vital for sustained weight loss.

Strategies to Cultivate Positivity

- **Daily Affirmations:** As mentioned earlier, daily affirmations can significantly impact your mindset. Start each day by repeating positive statements about yourself and your weight loss journey.
- **Visualization:** Spend a few minutes each day visualizing your success. Picture yourself achieving your goals, feeling confident and healthy. Visualization can help keep you motivated and focused on your desired outcome.
- **Gratitude Journaling:** Keep a gratitude journal and write down three things you are grateful for each day. This practice shifts your focus from what's lacking to what's abundant in your life, fostering a positive mindset.
- **Surround Yourself with Positivity:** Surround yourself with people who uplift and support you. Limit time with those who are negative or unsupportive. Engage with content that inspires and motivates you, whether it's books, podcasts, or social media accounts.

Handling Negativity and Setbacks

Positivity doesn't mean ignoring the challenges or setbacks you may encounter. It's about how you handle them. When faced with a setback, avoid self-blame and instead view it as a learning opportunity. Ask yourself:

- **What can I learn from this experience?**
- **How can I do things differently next time?**
- **What steps can I take to prevent this setback in the future?**

Maintaining a growth mindset, where you see challenges as opportunities for growth, can significantly enhance your ability to stay positive and motivated.

3. The Power of Self-Compassion

Understanding Self-Compassion

Self-compassion involves treating yourself with the same kindness and understanding you would offer a friend. Many people struggling with weight issues are often their harshest critics, leading to feelings of hopelessness and despair. Practicing self-compassion can help mitigate these negative emotions and provide a more supportive and nurturing environment for change.

Components of Self-Compassion

According to Dr. Kristin Neff, a leading researcher in self-compassion, there are three main components:

- **Self-Kindness:** Being warm and understanding toward yourself, especially in instances of pain or failure, rather than being harshly self-critical.
- **Common Humanity:** Recognizing that suffering and personal inadequacy are part of the shared human experience – something we all go through rather than something that happens to "me" alone.
- **Mindfulness:** Holding your painful thoughts and feelings in balanced awareness rather than over-identifying with them.

Practicing Self-Compassion

To cultivate self-compassion, start by acknowledging your struggles without judgment. When you notice self-critical thoughts, pause and consider how you would respond to a friend in a similar situation. Offer yourself words of comfort and encouragement.

Engage in self-care practices that nurture your body and mind. This could include activities like taking a relaxing bath, enjoying a hobby, or practicing mindfulness meditation. Remember, taking care of yourself is not indulgent but necessary for your overall well-being.

4. Setting Realistic Goals

The Importance of Goal Setting

Setting goals is essential for providing direction and motivation on your weight loss journey. However, it's crucial to set realistic and achievable goals to avoid frustration and discouragement. Unrealistic goals can set you up for failure, whereas realistic goals provide a clear path to success and allow for consistent progress.

SMART Goals

SMART goals are Specific, Measurable, Achievable, Relevant, and Time-bound. This framework ensures that your goals are clear and reachable. Here's how to apply SMART criteria to your weight loss goals:

- **Specific:** Clearly define what you want to achieve. Instead of saying, "I want to lose weight," specify, "I want to lose 10 pounds."
- **Measurable:** Ensure your goal can be tracked and measured. For example, "I will track my weight and measurements weekly."
- **Achievable:** Set goals that are challenging yet attainable. Losing 1-2 pounds per week is a healthy and achievable target.
- **Relevant:** Make sure your goals align with your broader objectives and values. Ask yourself, "Why is this goal important to me?"
- **Time-bound:** Set a timeframe for achieving your goal. For example, "I will lose 10 pounds in three months."

Breaking Down Larger Goals

Large goals can often feel overwhelming. Break them down into smaller, manageable steps to make them more attainable. For example, if your goal is to lose 50 pounds, break it down into increments of 5 or 10 pounds. Celebrate each milestone to stay motivated and encouraged.

Creating an Action Plan

Once you have your SMART goals, develop an action plan outlining the steps you need to take to achieve them. Your plan might include:

- **Dietary Changes:** Planning healthy meals, reducing portion sizes, or cutting back on sugar.
- **Exercise Routine:** Incorporating regular physical activity that you enjoy.
- **Support System:** Seeking support from friends, family, or a weight loss group.
- **Monitoring Progress:** Keeping track of your progress through a journal or app.

Revisit and adjust your action plan as needed to stay on track and make necessary adjustments.

Staying Committed

Consistency is key to achieving your weight loss goals. It's important to stay committed to your plan, even when progress seems slow. Remind yourself of your reasons for wanting to lose weight and keep your goals visible to maintain focus. Whether it's a vision board, a daily journal, or reminders on your phone, having constant reminders of your goals can help keep you motivated.

Dealing with Setbacks

Setbacks are a natural part of any journey. When they occur, it's essential not to let them derail your progress. Instead, view them as learning opportunities. Reflect on what led to the setback and how you can prevent it in the future. Be kind to yourself and recommit to your goals.

By focusing on these foundational aspects of mindset, you set the stage for a successful weight loss journey. Addressing and transforming limiting beliefs, cultivating positivity, practicing self-compassion, and setting realistic goals are crucial steps in ensuring that you are mentally prepared for the challenges ahead. Each subsequent chapter will build on this foundation, providing practical strategies and tools to help you achieve lasting success in your weight loss journey.

2

———

NUTRITION BASICS

1. Understanding Macronutrients

The Role of Macronutrients

Macronutrients are the nutrients our bodies need in large amounts to function correctly. They provide the energy necessary for growth, metabolism, and other bodily functions. The three primary macronutrients are carbohydrates, proteins, and fats. Each plays a unique role in the body, and understanding their functions is crucial for effective weight management.

- **Carbohydrates:** Often the primary source of energy, carbohydrates are broken down into glucose, which fuels our muscles and brain. They can be found in foods like grains, fruits, vegetables, and legumes. There are two main types of carbohydrates: simple and complex. Simple carbohydrates, like sugars, provide quick energy but can lead to spikes in blood sugar levels. Complex carbohydrates, found in whole grains and vegetables, provide sustained energy and are high in fiber.

- **Proteins:** Proteins are essential for building and repairing tissues, including muscles. They are made up of amino acids, some of which the body cannot produce on its own and must be obtained from food. Sources of protein include meat, fish, eggs, dairy products, legumes, and nuts. Protein also plays a role in satiety, helping you feel full and reducing overall calorie intake.

- **Fats:** Fats are necessary for absorbing fat-soluble vitamins (A, D, E, and K), protecting organs, and providing a concentrated source of energy. There are several types of fats, including saturated, unsaturated, and trans fats. Healthy fats, such as those found in avocados, nuts, seeds, and olive oil, support heart health and should be included in a balanced diet. Trans fats and excessive saturated fats, commonly found in processed foods, should be limited as they can contribute to heart disease and other health issues.

Balancing Macronutrients

A balanced diet includes appropriate portions of each macronutrient to meet your body's needs. The ideal macronutrient ratio can vary based on individual goals, activity levels, and metabolic health. However, a general guideline might be:

- **Carbohydrates:** 45-65% of daily calorie intake
- **Proteins:** 10-35% of daily calorie intake
- **Fats:** 20-35% of daily calorie intake

Tracking your macronutrient intake can help ensure you're getting the right balance. Apps and online tools can assist with this, providing personalized recommendations based on your specific needs.

Common Misconceptions about Macronutrients

- **Carbs are bad for you:** Carbohydrates are essential for energy, especially for brain function. It's the type and quantity of carbs that matter. Focus on whole, unprocessed carbs rather than refined sugars and flours.
- **All fats are unhealthy:** Healthy fats are crucial for overall health. It's important to choose unsaturated fats and limit trans fats and excessive saturated fats.
- **More protein is always better:** While protein is important, excessive intake can strain the kidneys and lead to imbalances. It's about finding the right amount for your body and goals.

2. The Role of Micronutrients

Understanding Micronutrients

Micronutrients are vitamins and minerals that our bodies require in smaller amounts but are nonetheless crucial for proper functioning. They support a wide range of physiological functions, including immune system performance, bone health, and energy production.

- **Vitamins:** These organic compounds are necessary for various biochemical processes. Key vitamins include Vitamin C (important for immune function), Vitamin D (crucial for bone health), and B Vitamins (important for energy metabolism).
- **Minerals:** Inorganic elements like calcium, potassium, iron, and magnesium are essential for processes such as bone formation, muscle contraction, and oxygen transport in the blood.

Sources of Micronutrients

Micronutrients are best obtained from a varied diet rich in fruits, vegetables, whole grains, lean proteins, and healthy fats. Each food group provides different vitamins and minerals:

- **Fruits and Vegetables:** Rich in vitamins A, C, E, and K, as well as folate, potassium, and magnesium.

- **Whole Grains:** Provide B vitamins, iron, magnesium, and fiber.
- **Proteins:** Meat, fish, dairy, and legumes are excellent sources of iron, zinc, and B vitamins.
- **Healthy Fats:** Nuts, seeds, and oils are good sources of Vitamin E and essential fatty acids.

Micronutrient Deficiencies

Deficiencies in micronutrients can lead to various health issues. Common deficiencies include:

- **Vitamin D:** Can lead to bone issues like osteoporosis.
- **Iron:** Can cause anemia, characterized by fatigue and weakness.
- **Vitamin B12:** Essential for nerve function and red blood cell production; deficiency can lead to neurological issues and anemia.

Ensuring a varied and balanced diet can help prevent these deficiencies. In some cases, supplementation may be necessary, especially for individuals with specific dietary restrictions or health conditions.

Debunking Myths about Micronutrients

- **More is always better:** Excessive intake of certain vitamins and minerals can be harmful. For example, too much Vitamin A can cause liver damage, and excessive iron can be toxic.

- **Supplements can replace a healthy diet:**
  While supplements can help address
  deficiencies, they cannot replace the array of
  nutrients provided by a varied, whole-food
  diet.

3. Debunking Diet Myths

Common Diet Myths

There are numerous myths about dieting that can lead
to confusion and frustration. Understanding the facts
can help you make informed decisions about your
nutrition.

- **Myth: Carbs make you fat:** Carbohydrates
  themselves are not fattening. It's the type and
  quantity that matter. Whole grains, fruits, and
  vegetables are nutrient-dense and can be part
  of a healthy diet.
- **Myth: Eating fat makes you fat:** Healthy fats
  are essential for your body. The key is to
  consume the right kinds of fats and in
  appropriate amounts.
- **Myth: Skipping meals helps you lose weight:**
  Skipping meals can lead to overeating later
  and can negatively impact your metabolism.
  Regular, balanced meals are more effective for
  weight management.
- **Myth: You need to detox:** Your body has its
  own detoxification systems, primarily the liver
  and kidneys. Eating a balanced diet, staying

hydrated, and getting regular exercise are the best ways to support these systems.

Fad Diets vs. Sustainable Eating

Fad diets often promise quick results but are typically unsustainable and can be harmful. Examples include extremely low-calorie diets, single-food diets, or eliminating entire food groups without medical reasons.

- **Extreme Calorie Restriction:** Severely limiting calories can lead to nutrient deficiencies, muscle loss, and metabolic slowdown.
- **Eliminating Food Groups:** Unless you have a medical condition, eliminating entire food groups (like carbs or fats) can lead to imbalances and nutrient deficiencies.
- **Single-Food Diets:** Diets that focus on one type of food (like the cabbage soup diet) are nutritionally incomplete and unsustainable.

Instead, focus on sustainable eating patterns that promote long-term health. This includes a balanced diet with a variety of foods, mindful eating, and regular physical activity.

The Importance of Individualized Nutrition

Nutrition is not one-size-fits-all. Factors like age, gender, activity level, metabolic health, and personal preferences all influence dietary needs. It's important to tailor your nutrition plan to your specific needs and goals.

Consider consulting a registered dietitian or nutritionist who can provide personalized advice and help you develop a balanced, sustainable eating plan that works for you.

4. Creating a Balanced Meal Plan

Principles of a Balanced Meal Plan

Creating a balanced meal plan involves including a variety of foods that provide all the necessary nutrients your body needs. Key principles include:

- **Variety:** Incorporate different foods from all food groups to ensure a wide range of nutrients.
- **Balance:** Ensure that meals contain a good mix of carbohydrates, proteins, and fats.
- **Moderation:** Pay attention to portion sizes and avoid overconsumption of any one type of food.

Meal Planning Strategies

- **Plan Ahead:** Take time each week to plan your meals and snacks. This can help you make healthier choices and avoid last-minute unhealthy options.

- **Prep in Advance:** Prepare ingredients or entire meals in advance to save time during the week. This can include chopping vegetables, cooking grains, or portioning out snacks.
- **Incorporate Leftovers:** Use leftovers creatively to reduce waste and save time. For example, use leftover roasted vegetables in a salad or stir-fry.

Sample Balanced Meal Plan

Here's an example of a balanced meal plan for a day:

- **Breakfast:** Greek yogurt with mixed berries, a sprinkle of granola, and a drizzle of honey.
- **Snack:** A handful of almonds and an apple.
- **Lunch:** Quinoa salad with mixed greens, cherry tomatoes, cucumber, chickpeas, feta cheese, and a lemon-tahini dressing.
- **Snack:** Carrot sticks with hummus.
- **Dinner:** Grilled salmon with roasted sweet potatoes and steamed broccoli.
- **Dessert:** A small piece of dark chocolate and a handful of fresh raspberries.

Adjusting Your Meal Plan

Your meal plan should be flexible and adjustable based on your needs and preferences. Listen to your body's hunger and fullness cues, and make adjustments as necessary. If you find certain meals or foods don't satisfy you, experiment with different options to find what works best.

By understanding the basics of nutrition, including macronutrients, micronutrients, and debunking common diet myths, you can create a balanced meal plan that supports your weight loss journey. This foundation of knowledge will empower you to make informed decisions about your diet and develop healthy eating habits that are sustainable in the long term. The next chapters will build on this knowledge, providing additional strategies and tools to help you achieve your weight loss goals.

3

EMOTIONAL EATING

1. Recognizing Emotional Triggers

Understanding Emotional Eating

Emotional eating refers to the tendency to consume food in response to emotions rather than hunger. Many people turn to food for comfort, stress relief, or as a reward. This behavior can lead to overeating, weight gain, and feelings of guilt and shame, which can perpetuate the cycle of emotional eating.

Common Emotional Triggers

To effectively manage emotional eating, it's crucial to identify the triggers that lead to this behavior. Common emotional triggers include:

- **Stress:** Work pressures, financial worries, and personal conflicts can lead to stress-induced eating.

- **Boredom:** Lack of engagement or stimulation can prompt mindless snacking.
- **Loneliness:** Feeling isolated or disconnected can drive individuals to seek comfort in food.
- **Sadness:** Depression or feelings of sadness can lead to overeating as a way to temporarily alleviate emotional pain.
- **Celebration:** Associating food with positive events can also be a trigger, leading to overeating during celebrations or social gatherings.

Self-Monitoring and Journaling

One effective way to identify emotional triggers is through self-monitoring and journaling. Keep a food diary where you log not only what you eat but also your emotions and circumstances surrounding each eating episode. Note the following:

- **Time and place:** When and where did the eating occur?
- **Emotions:** What were you feeling at the time? (e.g., stress, boredom, happiness)
- **Hunger levels:** Were you physically hungry or eating for emotional reasons?
- **Amount and type of food:** What and how much did you eat?

Reviewing your food diary can help you identify patterns and specific triggers that lead to emotional eating.

Mindfulness and Awareness

Practicing mindfulness can also help you become more aware of your emotional triggers. Mindfulness involves paying attention to your thoughts, feelings, and bodily sensations without judgment. When you feel the urge to eat, take a moment to pause and check in with yourself. Ask:

- **Am I truly hungry?**
- **What am I feeling right now?**
- **What do I need in this moment?**

This pause can help you distinguish between physical hunger and emotional needs, allowing you to make more conscious eating choices.

2. Strategies to Manage Cravings

Healthy Alternatives

When emotional cravings strike, it's essential to have healthier alternatives on hand. Here are some strategies to manage and satisfy cravings without derailing your weight loss efforts:

- **Nutrient-Dense Snacks:** Opt for snacks that provide nutritional value, such as fresh fruits, vegetables with hummus, nuts, or yogurt.

These options can satisfy your cravings while supporting your health goals.

- **Hydration:** Sometimes, thirst is mistaken for hunger. Drink a glass of water and wait a few minutes to see if the craving subsides.
- **Portion Control:** If you indulge in a treat, practice portion control to avoid overeating. Pre-portion snacks into single servings to prevent mindless munching.

Distraction Techniques

Distracting yourself from cravings can help reduce the urge to eat emotionally. Engage in activities that occupy your mind and hands, such as:

- **Physical Activity:** Go for a walk, do a workout, or practice yoga. Exercise can boost your mood and reduce stress, diminishing the desire to eat emotionally.
- **Hobbies:** Engage in hobbies that you enjoy, such as reading, crafting, playing an instrument, or gardening. These activities can shift your focus away from food.
- **Social Connection:** Reach out to a friend or family member for a chat. Social interaction can provide emotional support and reduce feelings of loneliness or boredom.

Mindful Eating Practices

Mindful eating involves paying full attention to the experience of eating, savoring each bite, and recognizing hunger and fullness cues. Practice mindful eating by:

- **Eating Slowly:** Take your time to chew thoroughly and enjoy the flavors and textures of your food.
- **Eliminating Distractions:** Avoid eating while watching TV, using your phone, or working. Focus solely on your meal.
- **Listening to Your Body:** Pay attention to your body's signals of hunger and fullness. Stop eating when you feel satisfied, not stuffed.

3. Developing Healthy Coping Mechanisms

Stress Reduction Techniques

Finding healthy ways to manage stress can reduce the reliance on food for emotional relief. Incorporate stress reduction techniques into your daily routine, such as:

- **Deep Breathing:** Practice deep breathing exercises to calm your mind and body. Inhale deeply through your nose, hold for a few seconds, and exhale slowly through your mouth.
- **Progressive Muscle Relaxation:** Tense and then relax each muscle group in your body, starting from your toes and working up to

your head. This technique can help alleviate physical tension and stress.

- **Mindfulness Meditation:** Set aside time each day for mindfulness meditation. Focus on your breath, sensations, or a guided meditation to promote relaxation and reduce stress.

Emotional Expression

Expressing your emotions in healthy ways can prevent them from building up and leading to emotional eating. Consider these outlets for emotional expression:

- **Journaling:** Write about your thoughts and feelings in a journal. This practice can help you process emotions and gain insight into your triggers.
- **Creative Arts:** Engage in creative activities such as drawing, painting, or writing. Creative expression can be therapeutic and provide an emotional release.
- **Talking:** Share your feelings with a trusted friend, family member, or therapist. Talking about your emotions can provide relief and support.

Building Resilience

Building emotional resilience involves developing the ability to bounce back from challenges and cope effectively with stress. Strengthening your resilience can reduce the likelihood of turning to food for comfort. Strategies include:

- **Positive Thinking:** Cultivate a positive mindset by focusing on your strengths, accomplishments, and potential. Practice gratitude and affirmations to reinforce positivity.
- **Problem-Solving Skills:** Enhance your problem-solving abilities by breaking down challenges into manageable steps. Develop a plan of action and take proactive steps to address issues.
- **Self-Care:** Prioritize self-care activities that nourish your body, mind, and spirit. This could include exercise, relaxation, hobbies, and social connections.

4. Building a Support System

Seeking Support from Loved Ones

Building a support system of friends and family can provide encouragement, accountability, and emotional support throughout your weight loss journey. Here's how to enlist their support:

- **Communicate Your Goals:** Share your weight loss goals and reasons with your loved ones. Explain how they can support you, whether through encouragement, joining you in healthy activities, or refraining from offering tempting foods.

- **Ask for Accountability:** Ask a friend or family member to be your accountability partner. Check in regularly to share progress, setbacks, and goals. Accountability can help keep you on track and motivated.
- **Participate in Activities Together:** Engage in healthy activities with your support system, such as cooking nutritious meals, exercising, or attending wellness events. Doing things together can strengthen your bond and make the journey more enjoyable.

Joining Support Groups

Support groups can provide a sense of community and understanding, especially for those dealing with similar challenges. Consider joining a weight loss support group, whether in-person or online. Benefits of support groups include:

- **Shared Experiences:** Hearing others' stories and experiences can provide insight, motivation, and reassurance that you're not alone.
- **Practical Advice:** Support groups often share practical tips and strategies for overcoming challenges and achieving success.

- **Emotional Support:** Connecting with others who understand your struggles can provide emotional support and encouragement.

Professional Help

Seeking professional help from a therapist, nutritionist, or weight loss coach can provide personalized guidance and support. Professionals can help you address emotional eating, develop healthy habits, and stay accountable. Consider the following options:

- **Therapist:** A therapist can help you explore the emotional and psychological aspects of your relationship with food. They can provide strategies for managing stress, coping with emotions, and building resilience.
- **Nutritionist:** A nutritionist can help you develop a balanced and sustainable meal plan that meets your nutritional needs and supports your weight loss goals.
- **Weight Loss Coach:** A weight loss coach can provide personalized guidance, motivation, and accountability. They can help you set realistic goals, develop an action plan, and stay on track.

Online Communities and Resources

Online communities and resources can offer additional support, motivation, and information. Join online forums, social media groups, or weight loss apps to connect with others on a similar journey. Benefits include:

- **24/7 Support:** Online communities are available around the clock, providing support and encouragement whenever you need it.
- **Diverse Perspectives:** Online communities offer a wide range of perspectives, experiences, and strategies, allowing you to learn from others and find what works best for you.
- **Resources and Tools:** Many online communities and apps provide resources such as meal plans, workout routines, tracking tools, and educational content.

By recognizing emotional triggers, managing cravings, developing healthy coping mechanisms, and building a support system, you can effectively address emotional eating and create a more balanced relationship with food. These strategies, combined with the foundational mindset shift from Chapter 1, will empower you to make lasting changes and achieve your weight loss goals.

4

EXERCISE ESSENTIALS

1. Finding the Right Exercise for You

Understanding the Importance of Exercise

Exercise plays a vital role in weight loss and overall health. Regular physical activity helps burn calories, improves cardiovascular health, builds muscle mass, and enhances mood. Finding the right exercise that you enjoy and can sustain is crucial for long-term success.

Types of Exercise

There are various types of exercises to choose from, and understanding the benefits of each can help you decide which ones to incorporate into your routine. The main types include:

- **Aerobic Exercise:** Activities like walking, running, swimming, and cycling fall under

aerobic exercise. These exercises increase
your heart rate and improve cardiovascular
health.

- **Strength Training:** This includes
  weightlifting, resistance band exercises, and
  bodyweight exercises like push-ups and
  squats. Strength training builds muscle mass,
  which can boost your metabolism.
- **Flexibility Exercises:** Activities such as yoga
  and stretching improve flexibility, reduce the
  risk of injury, and enhance overall physical
  performance.
- **Balance Exercises:** Balance-focused exercises,
  like tai chi or specific yoga poses, improve
  stability and coordination, which can be
  particularly beneficial as you age.

Assessing Your Fitness Level

Before starting any exercise program, it's important to
assess your current fitness level. This will help you set
realistic goals and choose appropriate activities.
Consider the following steps:

- **Consult with a Doctor:** Especially if you have
  any pre-existing conditions or haven't been
  active for a while, it's important to get medical
  clearance.
- **Fitness Assessment:** Conduct a basic fitness
  assessment to determine your current level.
  This can include measuring your resting heart

rate, doing a timed walk or run, and assessing your strength and flexibility.
- **Set Initial Goals:** Based on your assessment, set initial fitness goals. These should be realistic and tailored to your current abilities.

Finding Activities You Enjoy

The key to sticking with an exercise routine is to find activities you enjoy. If you dislike running, forcing yourself to do it won't be sustainable. Consider trying a variety of activities to see what you enjoy most. Some ideas include:

- **Walking or Hiking:** These are low-impact activities that can be done almost anywhere.
- **Dancing:** Join a dance class or follow along with online videos.
- **Swimming:** A great full-body workout that is easy on the joints.
- **Group Sports:** Join a local sports league or pick-up games for a fun, social way to exercise.
- **Fitness Classes:** Try classes like Zumba, spinning, or kickboxing to see what you enjoy.

2. Incorporating Movement into Daily Life

The Benefits of Daily Movement

While structured exercise sessions are important, incorporating movement throughout your day can significantly boost your overall activity level and help with weight loss. Small changes can add up and make a big difference over time.

Practical Tips for Increasing Daily Movement

- **Take the Stairs:** Opt for stairs instead of elevators whenever possible.
- **Walk or Bike to Work:** If feasible, walk or bike to work instead of driving.
- **Stand and Move at Work:** Use a standing desk, take regular breaks to stretch, or walk during phone calls.
- **Active Socializing:** Plan active outings with friends and family, such as hiking, playing sports, or going for a walk.
- **Household Chores:** Engage in activities like gardening, cleaning, or washing the car to get moving.

Using Technology to Stay Active

There are various apps and gadgets designed to help you stay active and track your progress. Consider the following:

- **Fitness Trackers:** Devices like Fitbit or Apple Watch can track your steps, workouts, and overall activity levels.
- **Activity Apps:** Apps like MyFitnessPal, Nike Training Club, or even simple step-tracking apps can help you stay motivated and on track.

- **Virtual Workouts:** Online workout platforms like Peloton, Beachbody On Demand, or free YouTube channels offer a wide variety of exercise classes you can do at home.

3. Strength Training vs. Cardio

The Benefits of Strength Training

Strength training is essential for building muscle mass, which can increase your metabolic rate and help you burn more calories at rest. Other benefits include:

- **Improved Muscle Tone:** Regular strength training helps define and tone your muscles.
- **Bone Health:** Weight-bearing exercises strengthen bones and reduce the risk of osteoporosis.
- **Increased Strength:** Everyday activities become easier as your strength improves.
- **Enhanced Metabolic Rate:** More muscle mass means a higher resting metabolic rate, helping you burn more calories throughout the day.

The Benefits of Cardio

Cardiovascular exercise, also known as aerobic exercise, is crucial for heart health and overall fitness. Benefits include:

- **Improved Heart Health:** Cardio exercises strengthen your heart and improve circulation.
- **Weight Loss:** Cardio workouts burn a significant amount of calories, aiding in weight loss.
- **Enhanced Endurance:** Regular cardio increases your stamina and energy levels.
- **Mental Health Benefits:** Aerobic exercise releases endorphins, which can improve mood and reduce stress.

Finding a Balance

Both strength training and cardio are important for a well-rounded fitness routine. Aim to incorporate both types of exercise into your weekly schedule. For example:

- **Strength Training:** Aim for at least two days per week. Focus on different muscle groups to allow for recovery.
- **Cardio:** Aim for at least 150 minutes of moderate-intensity cardio or 75 minutes of high-intensity cardio per week. This can be spread out across several days.

4. Creating a Sustainable Exercise Routine

Setting Realistic Exercise Goals

To create a sustainable exercise routine, it's important to set realistic goals that fit your lifestyle. Consider the following:

- **Start Small:** If you're new to exercise, start with shorter sessions and gradually increase the duration and intensity.
- **Be Consistent:** Aim for consistency rather than perfection. It's better to do shorter, regular workouts than sporadic long sessions.
- **Mix It Up:** Vary your workouts to keep things interesting and prevent boredom. This can also help prevent overuse injuries.

Building Your Routine

A well-rounded exercise routine should include a mix of cardio, strength training, and flexibility exercises. Here's a sample weekly plan:

- **Monday:** 30 minutes of moderate-intensity cardio (e.g., brisk walking or cycling)
- **Tuesday:** 30 minutes of strength training (e.g., full-body workout)
- **Wednesday:** Rest or active recovery (e.g., light stretching or yoga)
- **Thursday:** 30 minutes of high-intensity interval training (HIIT)
- **Friday:** 30 minutes of strength training (e.g., focusing on different muscle groups from Tuesday)

- **Saturday:** 30-60 minutes of low-intensity cardio (e.g., hiking or swimming)
- **Sunday:** Rest or active recovery (e.g., gentle yoga or a leisurely walk)

Staying Motivated

Maintaining motivation is key to sustaining your exercise routine. Here are some tips:

- **Set Short-Term Goals:** In addition to your long-term goals, set short-term goals to stay motivated. For example, aim to increase your weights every few weeks or run a 5K.
- **Track Your Progress:** Keep a workout journal or use an app to track your progress. Seeing your improvements can be very motivating.
- **Find a Workout Buddy:** Exercising with a friend can make workouts more enjoyable and hold you accountable.
- **Reward Yourself:** Treat yourself to non-food rewards when you reach your fitness goals. This could be a new workout outfit, a massage, or a fun outing.

Listening to Your Body

It's important to listen to your body and avoid overtraining. Signs of overtraining include persistent fatigue, decreased performance, and increased susceptibility to illness. Ensure you're getting enough rest and recovery between workouts, and don't be afraid to take a break if needed.

By understanding the importance of exercise and finding activities you enjoy, incorporating movement into daily life, balancing strength training and cardio, and creating a sustainable routine, you can make exercise an integral part of your weight loss journey. The next chapter will focus on breaking through plateaus and staying motivated to keep progressing toward your goals.

5

BREAKING THROUGH PLATEAUS

1. Understanding Weight Loss Plateaus

What is a Weight Loss Plateau?

A weight loss plateau occurs when your progress stalls despite maintaining your diet and exercise routine. This can be a frustrating experience, but it is a normal part of the weight loss process. Plateaus can last from a few weeks to several months and can be caused by various factors including metabolic adaptation, changes in water retention, and hormonal fluctuations.

The Science Behind Plateaus

As you lose weight, your body requires fewer calories to function, leading to a slower metabolism. This metabolic adaptation is a survival mechanism that helps your body conserve energy. Additionally, as you lose fat, your body composition changes, which can also impact your metabolic rate.

Common Causes of Plateaus

- **Caloric Deficit Adjustment:** As your weight decreases, your caloric needs also decrease. What was once a caloric deficit can become maintenance.
- **Loss of Lean Muscle Mass:** Muscle mass is metabolically active, and losing muscle can reduce your metabolic rate.
- **Dietary Habits:** Over time, you might unintentionally start consuming more calories or becoming less diligent with portion sizes.
- **Exercise Routine:** Your body can become efficient at your regular exercise routine, burning fewer calories than it did initially.

2. Adjusting Your Diet

Re-Evaluate Your Caloric Intake

As your body weight decreases, your daily caloric needs change. Use a calorie calculator to determine your new caloric requirements based on your current weight, age, sex, and activity level. Adjust your caloric intake accordingly to ensure you are maintaining a deficit.

Macronutrient Adjustment

Adjusting the balance of macronutrients—proteins, fats, and carbohydrates—can help break through a plateau. For instance, increasing your protein intake can help preserve lean muscle mass and boost your metabolic rate. Aim for a balanced diet with adequate protein, healthy fats, and complex carbohydrates.

Incorporate More Whole Foods

Refocus on whole, nutrient-dense foods that provide essential vitamins and minerals without excess calories. These foods can help you feel fuller longer and reduce the likelihood of overeating. Examples include:

- **Vegetables:** Leafy greens, cruciferous vegetables, bell peppers
- **Fruits:** Berries, apples, oranges
- **Whole Grains:** Quinoa, brown rice, oats
- **Lean Proteins:** Chicken breast, fish, legumes
- **Healthy Fats:** Avocado, nuts, seeds, olive oil

Avoid Hidden Calories

Be mindful of hidden calories in sauces, dressings, beverages, and snacks. These can add up quickly and impact your caloric deficit. Opt for homemade dressings, drink water or unsweetened beverages, and choose whole foods for snacks.

3. Modifying Your Exercise Routine

Incorporate Variety

Your body can adapt to a consistent exercise routine, making it less effective over time. Incorporating variety can help challenge your muscles and boost your metabolism. Try different types of exercise such as:

- **Strength Training:** Lifting weights, bodyweight exercises, resistance bands
- **Cardio:** Running, cycling, swimming, HIIT (High-Intensity Interval Training)
- **Flexibility and Balance:** Yoga, Pilates, stretching exercises

Increase Intensity

Increasing the intensity of your workouts can help you burn more calories and break through a plateau. This can be achieved by:

- **Adding Weight:** Increase the weight or resistance in your strength training exercises.
- **Increasing Speed:** Run or cycle faster.
- **Reducing Rest Time:** Shorten the rest periods between sets or exercises.

Focus on Strength Training

Building muscle through strength training can help boost your metabolism. Muscle tissue burns more calories at rest compared to fat tissue. Incorporate compound movements like squats, deadlifts, and bench presses, which engage multiple muscle groups.

Incorporate Interval Training

High-Intensity Interval Training (HIIT) involves short bursts of intense exercise followed by periods of rest or lower-intensity exercise. This type of training can help increase calorie burn and improve cardiovascular fitness. An example HIIT workout could be:

- 30 seconds of sprinting
- 1 minute of walking
- Repeat for 20-30 minutes

4. Staying Motivated

Revisit Your Goals

Plateaus can be discouraging, but revisiting your goals can help you stay motivated. Remind yourself why you started your weight loss journey and reflect on the progress you've made so far. Adjust your goals if necessary to keep them realistic and achievable.

Track Non-Scale Victories

Focusing solely on the scale can be disheartening during a plateau. Instead, track non-scale victories such as:

- **Improved Fitness Levels:** Increased strength, endurance, or flexibility
- **Clothing Fit:** Noticing that your clothes fit better or are becoming looser
- **Health Improvements:** Lower blood pressure, improved cholesterol levels, better blood sugar control
- **Energy Levels:** Feeling more energetic and less fatigued

Seek Support

Having a support system can make a significant difference in your motivation and accountability. Share your journey with friends, family, or join a weight loss group. Online communities and social media can also provide encouragement and tips from others who have faced similar challenges.

Celebrate Small Wins

Celebrate your achievements, no matter how small. Rewarding yourself for reaching milestones can help keep you motivated. Choose non-food rewards such as:

- **New Workout Gear:** Treat yourself to new exercise clothes or equipment.
- **Self-Care:** Enjoy a relaxing activity like a massage, spa day, or a hobby you love.
- **Experiences:** Plan a fun outing or activity that you enjoy.

Practice Patience and Persistence

Breaking through a plateau requires patience and persistence. Understand that weight loss is not a linear process and that plateaus are a normal part of the journey. Stay committed to your healthy habits, and trust that your efforts will eventually pay off.

In conclusion, breaking through a weight loss plateau involves understanding the underlying causes, making necessary adjustments to your diet and exercise routine, and maintaining motivation through realistic goal setting and support. By adopting a flexible and proactive approach, you can overcome plateaus and continue progressing toward your weight loss goals.

6

OVERCOMING MEDICAL AND GENETIC CHALLENGES

I. Understanding Metabolic Disorders

What Are Metabolic Disorders?

Metabolic disorders are conditions that disrupt normal metabolism, the process your body uses to convert food into energy. These disorders can affect how your body processes carbohydrates, fats, and proteins, leading to an imbalance that can hinder weight loss efforts. Common metabolic disorders include:

- **Hypothyroidism:** A condition where the thyroid gland doesn't produce enough thyroid hormones, slowing down metabolism.
- **Diabetes:** A chronic condition that affects how your body processes blood sugar (glucose).
- **Polycystic Ovary Syndrome (PCOS):** A hormonal disorder common among women of

reproductive age that can lead to weight gain
and difficulty losing weight.

Recognizing Symptoms

Recognizing the symptoms of metabolic disorders is crucial for early diagnosis and management. Symptoms can vary depending on the specific disorder but may include:

- **Fatigue and Weakness:** Persistent tiredness that doesn't improve with rest.
- **Unexplained Weight Gain:** Weight gain that occurs despite no changes in diet or exercise.
- **Cold Intolerance:** Feeling unusually cold, especially in the extremities.
- **Hair Loss and Dry Skin:** Symptoms often associated with thyroid disorders.
- **Irregular Menstrual Cycles:** Common in women with PCOS.

If you experience any of these symptoms, it's important to consult a healthcare professional for proper diagnosis and treatment.

Diagnosis and Treatment

Diagnosis of metabolic disorders typically involves a combination of medical history, physical examination, and laboratory tests. Blood tests can measure hormone levels, blood sugar, and other markers that indicate metabolic health. Once diagnosed, treatment may include:

- **Medication:** To manage symptoms and regulate metabolic processes.
- **Dietary Changes:** To support metabolic health and manage weight.
- **Exercise:** Regular physical activity tailored to individual needs.
- **Monitoring:** Regular follow-ups with healthcare providers to track progress and adjust treatment as necessary.

2. Working with Your Doctor

Finding the Right Healthcare Provider

Working with a healthcare provider who understands the complexities of weight loss and metabolic disorders is crucial. Look for a doctor who:

- **Specializes in Metabolic Health:** An endocrinologist or a specialist in metabolic disorders.
- **Takes a Holistic Approach:** Considers all aspects of your health, including diet, exercise, and mental well-being.
- **Communicates Clearly:** Explains medical conditions and treatment options in a way that you can understand and is open to answering your questions.

Preparing for Your Appointment

To make the most of your appointments, come prepared. Bring a list of your symptoms, medications, and any questions you have. Be honest about your lifestyle, diet, and exercise habits. This information helps your doctor provide the best possible care.

Developing a Treatment Plan

Work with your doctor to develop a personalized treatment plan. This plan should address:

- **Medical Management:** Medications and therapies to manage metabolic disorders.
- **Lifestyle Modifications:** Diet, exercise, and stress management strategies.
- **Regular Monitoring:** Follow-up appointments to track progress and make necessary adjustments.

3. Genetic Factors in Weight Loss

The Role of Genetics in Obesity

Genetics can play a significant role in an individual's propensity to gain weight and their ability to lose it. Some people may inherit genes that make them more susceptible to obesity. These genes can affect:

- **Appetite Regulation:** How your body signals hunger and fullness.

- **Metabolism:** How efficiently your body converts food into energy.
- **Fat Storage:** How and where your body stores fat.

Genetic Testing

Genetic testing can provide insights into your susceptibility to obesity and other metabolic conditions. While genetic testing is not necessary for everyone, it can be helpful if:

- **You Have a Family History of Obesity:** Understanding your genetic predisposition can help you tailor your weight loss approach.
- **You've Struggled with Weight Loss:** Despite following a healthy diet and exercise regimen.

Consult with your healthcare provider to determine if genetic testing is right for you.

Personalizing Your Approach

Understanding your genetic makeup can help you personalize your weight loss strategy. For example:

- **Diet:** Some people may benefit from specific dietary plans, such as a low-carb or Mediterranean diet, based on their genetic predisposition.

- **Exercise:** Tailor your exercise routine to your genetic profile, focusing on activities that are most effective for your body type.
- **Medical Interventions:** In some cases, medications or other medical interventions may be necessary to address genetic factors.

4. Tailoring Your Approach

Assessing Your Needs

Every individual is unique, and a one-size-fits-all approach to weight loss is rarely effective. Assess your needs by considering:

- **Medical History:** Any underlying medical conditions or metabolic disorders.
- **Genetic Factors:** Insights from genetic testing, if applicable.
- **Lifestyle:** Your daily habits, stress levels, and overall lifestyle.
- **Preferences:** Your dietary preferences and physical activity interests.

Creating a Personalized Strategy

Develop a weight loss plan that is tailored to your specific needs and preferences. This may include:

- **Customized Diet Plan:** Work with a nutritionist to develop a diet plan that suits your metabolic needs and preferences.

- **Exercise Routine:** Create an exercise routine that incorporates activities you enjoy and that are effective for your body type.
- **Behavioral Changes:** Implement strategies to manage stress, improve sleep, and build healthy habits.

Adapting as You Progress

Weight loss is a dynamic process, and your needs may change over time. Regularly reassess your progress and make adjustments as needed. This may involve:

- **Tweaking Your Diet:** Making changes to your diet based on your progress and any new insights from your healthcare provider.
- **Modifying Exercise Routine:** Adjusting your exercise routine to keep it challenging and enjoyable.
- **Addressing New Challenges:** As you progress, you may encounter new challenges that require adjustments to your plan.

Maintaining Flexibility

Flexibility is key to sustaining long-term weight loss. Be open to trying new strategies and making changes as needed. Listen to your body and work with your healthcare provider to ensure that your plan remains effective and sustainable.

. . .

Understanding and overcoming medical and genetic challenges is a critical component of successful weight loss. By recognizing and managing metabolic disorders, working closely with healthcare providers, and tailoring your approach to your unique needs, you can overcome these obstacles and achieve lasting success. Each subsequent chapter will build on this knowledge, providing additional strategies and tools to support your weight loss journey.

7

———

BUILDING HEALTHY HABITS

1. The Science of Habit Formation

Understanding Habits

Habits are the automatic routines and behaviors that we perform daily without much thought. They are formed through repetition and become ingrained in our brain's neural pathways. Understanding how habits are formed and how they function is essential for creating lasting change in your weight loss journey.

The Habit Loop

Charles Duhigg, in his book "The Power of Habit," describes the habit loop, which consists of three components:

- **Cue:** A trigger that initiates the behavior. This could be a specific time of day, an emotional state, or an environmental factor.

- **Routine:** The behavior itself, which can be positive or negative. For example, reaching for a snack when you're bored.
- **Reward:** The positive reinforcement that follows the behavior, making you more likely to repeat it. This could be the pleasure from eating a tasty treat or the relief from stress.

To build healthy habits, it's crucial to identify the cues and rewards associated with your existing habits and then modify the routines to align with your weight loss goals.

Creating New Habits

When creating new habits, start small and focus on consistency. Here are some steps to help you establish new, healthy routines:

- **Identify the Desired Behavior:** Clearly define the habit you want to establish. For example, "I want to eat a healthy breakfast every morning."
- **Choose a Cue:** Select a consistent cue to trigger the new habit. This could be something you already do regularly, like waking up or brushing your teeth.
- **Plan the Routine:** Decide on the specific actions you'll take as part of the new habit. For example, preparing a smoothie or oatmeal for breakfast.

- **Establish a Reward:** Choose a reward that will reinforce the new behavior. This could be something immediate, like enjoying a delicious meal, or long-term, like tracking your progress and seeing improvements in your health.

Maintaining Consistency

Consistency is key to forming new habits. Aim to perform the new behavior every day until it becomes automatic. Set reminders or use habit-tracking apps to help you stay on track. Be patient with yourself, as it can take several weeks to months for a new habit to become ingrained.

2. Small Changes, Big Results

The Power of Incremental Changes

Small, incremental changes can lead to significant, lasting results over time. Rather than attempting drastic transformations, focus on making manageable adjustments to your daily routines. These small changes can be easier to maintain and less overwhelming, leading to more sustainable weight loss.

Examples of Small Changes

- **Diet:** Start by adding more vegetables to your meals, replacing sugary drinks with water, or reducing portion sizes.

- **Exercise:** Begin with short, daily walks, take the stairs instead of the elevator, or incorporate a few minutes of stretching into your routine.
- **Lifestyle:** Go to bed 30 minutes earlier to improve sleep, practice mindfulness for a few minutes each day, or reduce screen time before bed.

Tracking Progress

Keep track of the small changes you're making and monitor your progress. Use a journal, app, or calendar to record your daily habits. Celebrate your successes, no matter how small, to stay motivated and acknowledge your progress.

3. Creating a Daily Routine

The Importance of Routine

Establishing a daily routine can provide structure and stability, making it easier to maintain healthy habits. A routine helps reduce decision fatigue, as you'll spend less time and energy deciding what to do each day. Instead, your healthy behaviors become part of your regular schedule.

Designing Your Routine

When designing your daily routine, consider the following:

- **Morning:** Start your day with healthy habits such as drinking water, eating a nutritious breakfast, and incorporating physical activity like stretching or a morning walk.
- **Afternoon:** Plan for a balanced lunch and include a mid-afternoon snack to keep your energy levels stable. Schedule regular breaks to move and stay active.
- **Evening:** Prepare a healthy dinner, limit screen time, and engage in relaxing activities to wind down. Establish a bedtime routine that promotes good sleep hygiene.

Flexibility and Adaptation

While routines are beneficial, it's also important to remain flexible and adapt to changes. Life can be unpredictable, and rigid routines can sometimes lead to frustration. Be prepared to adjust your routine as needed and have backup plans in place for maintaining your healthy habits.

4. Tracking Your Progress

The Benefits of Tracking

Tracking your progress is an effective way to stay motivated and hold yourself accountable. It provides tangible evidence of your efforts and helps you identify patterns, successes, and areas for improvement.

Methods of Tracking

There are various methods you can use to track your progress:

- **Journaling:** Keep a daily journal where you record your meals, exercise, and thoughts about your weight loss journey. Reflect on your achievements and challenges regularly.
- **Apps and Technology:** Utilize apps that track your food intake, physical activity, and weight loss progress. Many apps also offer features like reminders, goal setting, and community support.
- **Measurements:** Regularly measure and record your weight, body measurements, and other relevant metrics like body fat percentage or fitness levels.
- **Photos:** Take progress photos to visually document your changes. Comparing photos over time can be a powerful motivator.

Reflecting and Adjusting

Periodically review your tracking data to assess your progress and make any necessary adjustments to your plan. Celebrate your achievements, no matter how small, and use any setbacks as learning opportunities. Adjust your goals and strategies as needed to stay on track and continue progressing toward your long-term objectives.

. . .

By understanding the science of habit formation and focusing on building healthy habits, you create a strong foundation for sustainable weight loss. Implementing small changes, establishing a daily routine, and tracking your progress are essential strategies for maintaining motivation and achieving lasting success. Each subsequent chapter will continue to build on these principles, providing you with practical tools and strategies to support your weight loss journey.

8

THE IMPORTANCE OF SLEEP

1. The Sleep-Weight Connection

The Role of Sleep in Weight Management

Sleep is often overlooked in weight management, but it plays a crucial role in maintaining a healthy weight. Quality sleep affects various physiological processes, including metabolism, appetite regulation, and energy balance. Understanding the connection between sleep and weight is essential for anyone looking to lose weight or maintain a healthy weight.

Hormonal Influence

Two hormones, ghrelin and leptin, play a significant role in regulating hunger and satiety. Ghrelin stimulates appetite, while leptin signals to the brain that you are full. Lack of sleep increases ghrelin levels and decreases leptin levels, leading to increased hunger and reduced feelings of fullness. This hormonal imbalance can result in overeating and weight gain.

Impact on Metabolism

Sleep deprivation negatively affects your metabolism, making it more challenging to burn calories efficiently. Insufficient sleep can lead to insulin resistance, a condition where the body's cells become less responsive to insulin. This can result in higher blood sugar levels and increased fat storage, contributing to weight gain and increasing the risk of type 2 diabetes.

Behavioral Effects

Lack of sleep can also impact your behavior and decision-making abilities. When you are tired, you are more likely to make unhealthy food choices, such as reaching for high-calorie, sugary snacks for a quick energy boost. Additionally, sleep deprivation can reduce your motivation to exercise, further hindering your weight loss efforts.

2. Improving Sleep Quality

Establishing a Sleep Routine

A consistent sleep routine is essential for improving sleep quality. Aim to go to bed and wake up at the same time every day, even on weekends. This helps regulate your body's internal clock and promotes better sleep. Create a relaxing bedtime routine to signal to your body that it's time to wind down. This could include activities such as reading, taking a warm bath, or practicing meditation.

Creating a Sleep-Friendly Environment

Your sleep environment significantly impacts the quality of your sleep. Ensure your bedroom is conducive to sleep by:

- **Keeping it Dark:** Use blackout curtains or an eye mask to block out light.
- **Reducing Noise:** Use earplugs or a white noise machine to minimize disturbances.
- **Maintaining a Comfortable Temperature:** Keep your bedroom cool, ideally between 60-67°F (15-19°C).
- **Choosing the Right Mattress and Pillows:** Invest in a comfortable mattress and pillows that provide adequate support.

Limiting Stimulants

Avoid consuming stimulants such as caffeine and nicotine close to bedtime, as they can interfere with your ability to fall asleep. Be mindful of hidden sources of caffeine, such as certain teas, sodas, and chocolate. Additionally, limit alcohol intake, as it can disrupt your sleep cycle and reduce sleep quality.

Managing Light Exposure

Exposure to natural light during the day helps regulate your sleep-wake cycle. Spend time outside during daylight hours, especially in the morning. In the evening, limit exposure to blue light from screens (phones, tablets, computers) as it can interfere with melatonin production, the hormone that regulates sleep. Consider using blue light filters on your devices or wearing blue light-blocking glasses.

Incorporating Relaxation Techniques

Relaxation techniques can help calm your mind and prepare your body for sleep. Consider incorporating the following practices into your bedtime routine:

- **Deep Breathing:** Practice deep breathing exercises to reduce stress and promote relaxation.
- **Progressive Muscle Relaxation:** Tense and then relax each muscle group to release physical tension.
- **Guided Imagery:** Visualize a peaceful scene or experience to help calm your mind.
- **Mindfulness Meditation:** Focus on the present moment and let go of any racing thoughts.

3. Creating a Sleep-Friendly Environment

Optimizing Your Bedroom for Sleep

Your bedroom environment plays a crucial role in the quality of your sleep. Making your bedroom a sanctuary for rest can significantly improve your sleep quality. Here are some tips to optimize your sleep environment:

- **Keep it Cool:** A cooler room temperature, around 60-67°F (15-19°C), is ideal for sleep. Use fans, air conditioning, or breathable bedding to maintain a comfortable temperature.
- **Reduce Light Exposure:** Darkness signals your body that it's time to sleep. Use blackout curtains, shades, or an eye mask to block out light. Consider covering or removing electronic devices that emit light.
- **Minimize Noise:** Reduce noise pollution by using earplugs, white noise machines, or soundproofing your room. If you live in a noisy area, consider using heavy curtains or carpeting to dampen sound.
- **Choose Comfortable Bedding:** Invest in a good-quality mattress and pillows that provide the right support for your body. Your bedding should be comfortable and made of breathable materials.
- **Declutter Your Space:** A tidy bedroom can create a sense of calm and relaxation. Keep your bedroom clean and free of clutter to promote a peaceful environment.

Promoting a Relaxing Atmosphere

Creating a relaxing atmosphere in your bedroom can help signal to your body that it's time to wind down and prepare for sleep. Consider incorporating the following elements:

- **Aromatherapy:** Use essential oils such as lavender, chamomile, or cedarwood to create a calming environment. You can use a diffuser, pillow spray, or add a few drops to your bath.
- **Soft Lighting:** Use dim, warm lighting in the evening to create a relaxing ambiance. Avoid bright overhead lights and opt for bedside lamps or string lights.
- **Calming Colors:** Choose calming colors for your bedroom decor, such as soft blues, greens, or neutral tones. These colors can help create a soothing atmosphere.

Incorporating Technology Wisely

While technology can often disrupt sleep, there are ways to use it to your advantage. Here are some tips for incorporating technology wisely:

- **Sleep Apps:** Use sleep-tracking apps to monitor your sleep patterns and identify areas for improvement. Some apps also offer guided meditations, relaxation exercises, and white noise features.
- **Smart Lighting:** Consider using smart lighting systems that gradually dim in the evening and brighten in the morning to mimic natural light patterns.

- **Wearable Devices:** Wearable devices such as fitness trackers can provide insights into your sleep quality and patterns. Use this information to make adjustments to your sleep routine.

4. Managing Sleep Disorders

Recognizing Common Sleep Disorders

Sleep disorders can significantly impact your ability to get quality rest and, in turn, affect your weight management efforts. Common sleep disorders include:

- **Insomnia:** Difficulty falling asleep, staying asleep, or waking up too early and not being able to go back to sleep.
- **Sleep Apnea:** A condition where breathing repeatedly stops and starts during sleep, leading to disrupted sleep and poor oxygenation.
- **Restless Leg Syndrome (RLS):** An uncontrollable urge to move your legs, usually due to uncomfortable sensations, which can interfere with sleep.
- **Narcolepsy:** Excessive daytime sleepiness and sudden, uncontrollable episodes of falling asleep during the day.

Seeking Professional Help

If you suspect you have a sleep disorder, it's essential to seek professional help. A healthcare provider or sleep specialist can diagnose and treat sleep disorders. Treatment options may include:

- **Cognitive Behavioral Therapy for Insomnia (CBT-I):** A structured program that helps identify and change thoughts and behaviors that cause or worsen sleep problems.
- **Continuous Positive Airway Pressure (CPAP) Therapy:** A common treatment for sleep apnea that uses a machine to deliver a steady stream of air to keep the airways open during sleep.
- **Medications:** In some cases, medications may be prescribed to help manage sleep disorders. These should be used under the guidance of a healthcare provider.
- **Lifestyle Changes:** Incorporating healthy sleep habits, such as maintaining a consistent sleep schedule, reducing caffeine and alcohol intake, and creating a relaxing bedtime routine.

Implementing Lifestyle Changes

In addition to seeking professional help, making lifestyle changes can significantly improve sleep quality. Here are some strategies to consider:

- **Regular Exercise:** Engaging in regular physical activity can help regulate your sleep patterns and improve sleep quality. Aim for at least 30 minutes of moderate exercise most days of the week, but avoid vigorous exercise close to bedtime.
- **Healthy Diet:** Eating a balanced diet and avoiding heavy meals, caffeine, and alcohol close to bedtime can improve sleep quality. Consider incorporating sleep-promoting foods, such as those rich in magnesium and tryptophan, into your diet.
- **Stress Management:** Chronic stress can interfere with sleep. Practice stress management techniques, such as mindfulness meditation, yoga, or deep breathing exercises, to reduce stress and promote relaxation.

By prioritizing sleep and making necessary changes to improve sleep quality, you can enhance your overall well-being and support your weight management efforts. Quality sleep is a fundamental component of a healthy lifestyle and should not be overlooked.

9

___

STRESS MANAGEMENT

I. How Stress Affects Weight

The Connection Between Stress and Weight Gain

Stress is an often overlooked factor in weight management. When you experience stress, your body undergoes several physiological changes that can lead to weight gain. The hormone cortisol, also known as the stress hormone, plays a significant role in this process. During periods of stress, cortisol levels increase, which can lead to:

- **Increased Appetite:** High cortisol levels can boost your appetite, making you crave high-calorie, sugary foods.
- **Fat Storage:** Cortisol encourages the storage of fat, particularly around the abdomen, which is associated with greater health risks.

- **Metabolic Changes:** Stress can slow down your metabolism, making it harder to lose weight even if you are eating well and exercising regularly.

Understanding this connection is crucial because it highlights the importance of managing stress as part of a comprehensive weight loss plan.

Emotional Eating

Stress often leads to emotional eating, where food is used as a coping mechanism for dealing with negative emotions. This can create a vicious cycle: stress leads to overeating, which leads to weight gain and further stress. Identifying the triggers for emotional eating is the first step in breaking this cycle.

Sleep Disruption

Chronic stress can also disrupt your sleep patterns, leading to insomnia or poor-quality sleep. Poor sleep has been linked to weight gain, as it can affect the hormones that regulate hunger and appetite, leading to increased cravings for unhealthy foods.

2. Techniques for Stress Reduction

Mindfulness and Meditation

Mindfulness and meditation are powerful tools for managing stress. These practices help you become more aware of your thoughts and feelings, allowing you to respond to stress in a healthier way. Mindfulness involves paying attention to the present moment without judgment, while meditation involves focusing your mind on a particular object, thought, or activity to achieve a mentally clear and emotionally calm state.

- **Mindfulness Practices:** Simple mindfulness practices include mindful breathing, mindful eating, and body scan meditation. These practices can help reduce stress by bringing your focus back to the present moment and away from stress-inducing thoughts.
- **Meditation Techniques:** There are various types of meditation, including guided meditation, transcendental meditation, and loving-kindness meditation. Experiment with different techniques to find the one that works best for you.

Exercise

Physical activity is a proven stress reliever. Exercise helps lower cortisol levels and releases endorphins, which are natural mood boosters. Incorporating regular exercise into your routine can significantly reduce stress levels and improve your overall mental health.

- **Types of Exercise:** Both aerobic exercises (such as walking, running, or cycling) and

anaerobic exercises (such as strength training
or yoga) can be effective in managing stress.

- **Consistency:** Aim to incorporate at least 30
  minutes of physical activity into your daily
  routine. Even small amounts of exercise can
  make a difference in your stress levels.

Deep Breathing Exercises

Deep breathing exercises can quickly reduce stress and
promote relaxation. Techniques such as diaphragmatic
breathing, 4-7-8 breathing, and box breathing are
simple yet effective methods to calm your mind and
body.

- **Diaphragmatic Breathing:** Inhale deeply
  through your nose, allowing your abdomen to
  expand, and exhale slowly through your
  mouth.
- **4-7-8 Breathing:** Inhale for a count of 4, hold
  for a count of 7, and exhale for a count of 8.
- **Box Breathing:** Inhale for a count of 4, hold
  for a count of 4, exhale for a count of 4, and
  hold again for a count of 4.

Progressive Muscle Relaxation

Progressive muscle relaxation (PMR) involves tensing
and then relaxing different muscle groups in your
body. This technique can help reduce physical tension
associated with stress and promote a sense of calm.

- **How to Practice PMR:** Start with your toes and work your way up to your head. Tense each muscle group for a few seconds, then release and relax.

Creative Outlets

Engaging in creative activities can be a great way to manage stress. Whether it's painting, writing, playing music, or gardening, creative outlets provide an opportunity to express yourself and focus your mind on something enjoyable and fulfilling.

Social Support

Connecting with others can help alleviate stress. Whether it's talking to a friend, joining a support group, or participating in social activities, having a strong support network can provide emotional comfort and practical assistance in times of stress.

3. Incorporating Mindfulness and Meditation

Mindfulness in Daily Life

Integrating mindfulness into your daily routine can help you manage stress more effectively. Here are some simple ways to practice mindfulness throughout the day:

- **Mindful Eating:** Pay attention to the taste, texture, and aroma of your food. Eat slowly and savor each bite.

- **Mindful Walking:** Take a walk and focus on the sensation of your feet touching the ground, the sounds around you, and the feeling of the air on your skin.
- **Mindful Breathing:** Take a few moments throughout the day to focus on your breath. Notice the sensation of the air entering and leaving your body.

Developing a Meditation Practice

Starting a meditation practice doesn't require a lot of time or special equipment. Here are some tips to help you get started:

- **Find a Quiet Space:** Choose a quiet, comfortable place where you won't be disturbed.
- **Set a Timer:** Start with just a few minutes each day and gradually increase the time as you become more comfortable.
- **Focus on Your Breath:** Pay attention to your breathing, noticing the inhale and exhale. If your mind wanders, gently bring your focus back to your breath.
- **Use Guided Meditations:** There are many apps and online resources that offer guided meditations for beginners. These can be helpful in providing structure and guidance as you start your practice.

4. Creating a Relaxation Plan

Identifying Stress Triggers

The first step in creating a relaxation plan is to identify the specific stressors in your life. These could be work-related, family-related, or personal issues. Write down the main sources of stress and consider how they affect your daily life and well-being.

Developing Stress-Reduction Strategies

Once you've identified your stress triggers, develop a list of strategies to manage and reduce stress. These strategies might include:

- **Time Management:** Prioritize tasks and create a schedule to manage your time more effectively.
- **Healthy Lifestyle Choices:** Maintain a balanced diet, get regular exercise, and ensure you're getting enough sleep.
- **Relaxation Techniques:** Incorporate techniques such as deep breathing, meditation, and progressive muscle relaxation into your daily routine.
- **Social Support:** Reach out to friends, family, or support groups for emotional support and practical advice.

Creating a Daily Relaxation Routine

Establishing a daily relaxation routine can help you manage stress more effectively. Here's an example of what a relaxation routine might look like:

- **Morning:** Start your day with a few minutes of deep breathing or meditation to set a calm tone for the day.
- **Midday:** Take a short walk during your lunch break to clear your mind and reduce stress.
- **Evening:** Spend some time engaging in a relaxing activity such as reading, listening to music, or practicing a hobby.
- **Before Bed:** Practice a relaxation technique such as progressive muscle relaxation or guided imagery to help you unwind and prepare for sleep.

Monitoring and Adjusting Your Plan

Regularly review and adjust your relaxation plan to ensure it remains effective. Pay attention to how different strategies affect your stress levels and make changes as needed. Remember that managing stress is an ongoing process, and what works for you may change over time.

By understanding how stress affects your body and weight, and by implementing effective stress-reduction techniques, you can significantly enhance your weight loss efforts and overall well-being. Each subsequent chapter will build on this foundation, providing additional strategies and tools to help you achieve lasting success in your weight loss journey.

10

UNDERSTANDING METABOLISM

1. What is Metabolism?

Defining Metabolism

Metabolism encompasses all the chemical processes that occur within your body to maintain life. These processes convert the food you eat into energy, which fuels everything from breathing to exercising. Metabolism can be broadly divided into two categories:

- **Catabolism:** The process of breaking down molecules to obtain energy. For example, breaking down carbohydrates into glucose.
- **Anabolism:** The process of synthesizing all compounds needed by the cells. For example, building muscle proteins from amino acids.

Basal Metabolic Rate (BMR)

Your Basal Metabolic Rate (BMR) is the number of calories your body needs to perform basic life-sustaining functions, such as breathing, circulation, and cell production. BMR accounts for approximately 60-75% of the total calories you burn each day and is influenced by several factors, including age, gender, body composition, and genetics.

Total Daily Energy Expenditure (TDEE)

Total Daily Energy Expenditure (TDEE) includes your BMR plus the calories burned through physical activity, digestion, and other non-resting activities. Understanding your TDEE is essential for weight management, as it helps you determine how many calories you need to consume to maintain, lose, or gain weight.

2. Factors that Affect Metabolism

Age and Metabolism

As you age, your metabolism naturally slows down due to a decrease in muscle mass and hormonal changes. This can lead to weight gain if dietary and activity levels remain unchanged. Strategies to counteract this include engaging in regular strength training to preserve muscle mass and adjusting calorie intake.

Gender and Metabolism

Men typically have a higher BMR than women due to having more muscle mass, which burns more calories at rest. Women's metabolism can also be affected by hormonal changes throughout their menstrual cycle, pregnancy, and menopause.

Muscle Mass and Metabolism

Muscle tissue is more metabolically active than fat tissue, meaning it burns more calories at rest. Increasing your muscle mass through strength training can boost your BMR and help you burn more calories even when you're not exercising.

Genetics and Metabolism

Genetic factors can influence your metabolic rate and how efficiently your body processes food and converts it into energy. While you can't change your genetics, understanding your unique metabolic traits can help you tailor your diet and exercise plan more effectively.

Hormonal Influences

Hormones play a significant role in regulating metabolism. Thyroid hormones, for example, have a profound impact on metabolic rate. Conditions like hypothyroidism (low thyroid hormone levels) can slow metabolism, making weight loss more challenging. Other hormones, such as insulin, cortisol, and leptin, also influence appetite, energy storage, and metabolic rate.

3. Boosting Your Metabolic Rate

Regular Exercise

Engaging in regular physical activity, particularly a combination of aerobic (cardio) and anaerobic (strength training) exercises, can significantly boost your metabolic rate. Cardio exercises increase the number of calories burned during the activity, while strength training builds muscle mass, which enhances your resting metabolic rate.

High-Intensity Interval Training (HIIT)

HIIT involves short bursts of intense exercise followed by rest or low-intensity exercise. HIIT workouts can increase your metabolic rate for hours after the workout, a phenomenon known as excess post-exercise oxygen consumption (EPOC).

Eating Enough Protein

Protein has a higher thermic effect of food (TEF) compared to carbohydrates and fats, meaning it requires more energy to digest and process. Including adequate protein in your diet can boost your metabolism and help you feel full, reducing overall calorie intake.

Staying Hydrated

Drinking water can temporarily boost metabolism by about 24-30%. Cold water is particularly effective, as your body uses extra calories to heat the water to body temperature. Staying hydrated also helps your body perform its metabolic processes more efficiently.

Eating Small, Frequent Meals

Eating smaller, more frequent meals can help keep your metabolism active throughout the day. Avoiding long periods of fasting helps prevent your body from going into "starvation mode," where it conserves energy and reduces metabolic rate.

Getting Enough Sleep

Sleep is crucial for metabolic health. Lack of sleep can disrupt the hormones that regulate hunger and appetite, leading to increased calorie intake and weight gain. Aim for 7-9 hours of quality sleep per night to support a healthy metabolism.

4. Myths about Metabolism

Myth 1: Metabolism Alone Determines Weight Loss

While metabolism plays a significant role in weight management, it's not the only factor. Total calorie intake, physical activity, and other lifestyle factors also contribute to weight loss or gain. Focusing solely on boosting metabolism without considering other factors is unlikely to lead to significant weight loss.

Myth 2: Eating Certain Foods Can Dramatically Boost Metabolism

Certain foods, like green tea, chili peppers, and coffee, are often touted as metabolism boosters. While these foods may have a minor impact on metabolic rate, they are not magic bullets. Sustainable weight loss comes from a balanced diet and regular exercise rather than relying on specific foods to boost metabolism.

Myth 3: Skipping Meals Slows Down Your Metabolism

Skipping meals can lead to decreased energy levels and increased hunger, potentially causing overeating later in the day. However, the occasional skipped meal doesn't significantly slow down metabolism. What's more important is the overall pattern of eating and ensuring you get enough nutrients and calories throughout the day.

Myth 4: Thin People Have Faster Metabolisms

Body size and composition influence metabolic rate, but being thin doesn't necessarily mean having a faster metabolism. In fact, larger bodies often have higher metabolic rates because they require more energy to maintain. Muscle mass, activity level, and other factors are more significant determinants of metabolic rate.

Myth 5: You Can't Change Your Metabolism

While genetics play a role in determining metabolic rate, you can influence your metabolism through lifestyle changes. Building muscle mass, staying active, eating a balanced diet, and getting enough sleep can all contribute to a healthier metabolism.

By understanding the intricacies of metabolism, you can better tailor your weight loss strategy to your unique needs. Recognizing the factors that influence metabolism and adopting habits that support a healthy metabolic rate will help you achieve and maintain your weight loss goals more effectively. The subsequent chapters will continue to provide practical strategies and insights to help you navigate your weight loss journey with confidence and success.

11

SOCIAL INFLUENCES ON WEIGHT LOSS

I. Navigating Social Pressures

Understanding Social Influences

Social influences play a significant role in our behaviors and attitudes, including those related to weight and health. Friends, family, coworkers, and even societal norms can impact your weight loss journey, either positively or negatively. Recognizing these influences is crucial for navigating social pressures effectively.

Identifying Negative Influences

Negative social influences can come from various sources:

- **Family and Friends:** Well-meaning loved ones might unintentionally sabotage your efforts by encouraging unhealthy eating or

discouraging your exercise routines. They
might say things like, "Just have one piece of
cake" or "You're already fine the way you are;
you don't need to lose weight."

- **Work Environment:** Office culture often
includes unhealthy food options during
meetings, celebrations, and even regular
workdays. It can be challenging to resist these
temptations.
- **Social Gatherings:** Parties, holidays, and
other social events frequently revolve around
food and drink, making it difficult to stick to
your healthy habits.

Strategies to Navigate Social Pressures

- **Communicate Your Goals:** Let your friends
and family know about your weight loss goals
and how they can support you. Be clear about
what you need from them, whether it's
avoiding certain foods around you or joining
you in healthy activities.
- **Set Boundaries:** It's important to establish
boundaries when it comes to social situations.
Politely decline offers of unhealthy food and
explain your reasons. You might say, "I'm
focusing on my health right now, so I'll pass
on the cake, but thank you."
- **Bring Healthy Alternatives:** When attending
social events, bring a healthy dish to share.
This ensures there will be something

nutritious for you to eat and can also introduce others to healthier options.

- **Practice Assertiveness:** Learn to say no confidently and assertively. You don't have to justify your choices to others. A simple, "No, thank you," is sufficient.
- **Find Supportive Communities:** Surround yourself with like-minded individuals who support your goals. Join online forums, social media groups, or local weight loss groups where you can share experiences, gain advice, and receive encouragement.

2. Building a Support Network

The Importance of Support

A strong support network can make a significant difference in your weight loss journey. Supportive friends, family, and communities can provide encouragement, accountability, and motivation, helping you stay on track.

Types of Support

- **Emotional Support:** This includes encouragement, understanding, and empathy. Emotional support can help you stay positive and resilient, especially during challenging times.
- **Practical Support:** This involves tangible help, such as preparing healthy meals

together, joining you for workouts, or helping with childcare so you can exercise.

- **Informational Support:** Providing valuable information, advice, and resources can help you make informed decisions about your health and weight loss strategies.

Cultivating a Supportive Environment

- **Share Your Journey:** Open up to your close friends and family about your weight loss journey. Sharing your goals, challenges, and successes can help them understand your needs and offer better support.
- **Seek Professional Help:** Consider working with professionals such as nutritionists, personal trainers, or therapists. They can provide expert guidance and support tailored to your specific needs.
- **Join Support Groups:** Look for local or online support groups focused on weight loss and healthy living. These groups can provide a sense of community and belonging, helping you stay motivated and accountable.
- **Be a Role Model:** Inspire others by sharing your progress and healthy habits. This can create a ripple effect, encouraging those around you to adopt healthier lifestyles.

3. Dealing with Sabotage

Recognizing Sabotage

Sabotage can be subtle or overt, intentional or unintentional. It can come from others who may feel threatened by your changes, jealous of your progress, or simply uncomfortable with change. Common forms of sabotage include:

- **Encouraging Unhealthy Choices:** Offering you unhealthy foods or pressuring you to skip workouts.
- **Undermining Your Efforts:** Making negative comments about your progress or suggesting that your goals are unrealistic.
- **Disregarding Your Boundaries:** Ignoring your requests for support and continuing behaviors that hinder your progress.

Strategies to Handle Sabotage

- **Address the Issue:** Have an open and honest conversation with the person who is sabotaging you. Explain how their actions affect you and what you need from them to support your goals.
- **Stay Firm:** Stick to your boundaries and remind others of your commitment to your health. Be consistent in your responses to sabotage attempts.
- **Limit Exposure:** If certain individuals continually sabotage your efforts, consider

limiting your interactions with them. Surround yourself with positive influences instead.

- **Seek Support Elsewhere:** If you can't find support within your immediate circle, look for it in other areas. Join weight loss groups, find online communities, or work with professionals who can provide the encouragement and guidance you need.

4. Celebrating Your Successes

The Importance of Celebration

Celebrating your successes, both big and small, is crucial for maintaining motivation and recognizing your progress. Acknowledging your achievements reinforces positive behavior and helps you stay focused on your goals.

Ways to Celebrate

- **Non-Food Rewards:** Find non-food ways to reward yourself for your progress. This could include treating yourself to a new outfit, enjoying a spa day, or buying a book or gadget you've been wanting.
- **Share Your Success:** Share your achievements with your support network. Celebrating together can strengthen your relationships and provide additional encouragement.

- **Reflect on Your Journey:** Take time to reflect on how far you've come. Journaling about your experiences, challenges, and victories can help you appreciate your progress and stay motivated.
- **Set New Goals:** Use your achievements as a foundation for setting new goals. Continuous growth and progress keep you engaged and focused on your long-term objectives.

Maintaining a Positive Outlook

Staying positive throughout your weight loss journey is essential. Celebrate every step forward, no matter how small. Remember that progress is not always linear, and setbacks are a natural part of the process. By recognizing and celebrating your successes, you maintain a positive outlook and build the resilience needed to achieve your long-term goals.

Navigating social influences is a crucial aspect of your weight loss journey. By identifying and addressing negative influences, building a strong support network, handling sabotage effectively, and celebrating your successes, you create a supportive environment that fosters lasting change. Each of these strategies contributes to a positive and resilient mindset, essential for achieving and maintaining your weight loss goals.

12

———

THE ROLE OF TECHNOLOGY

1. Using Apps and Gadgets

Choosing the Right Apps

The digital age has brought an array of apps designed to help with weight loss. These apps can track calories, monitor physical activity, provide workout plans, and even offer psychological support. Here are some key types of apps to consider:

- **Calorie Counters:** MyFitnessPal, Lose It!, and Cronometer are popular choices. They allow you to log your food intake and track calories, nutrients, and more.
- **Fitness Trackers:** Apps like Fitbit, Strava, and MapMyRun can monitor your physical activity, including steps taken, calories burned, and exercise routines.

- **Meal Planning:** Apps such as Mealime, Paprika, and Yummly help you plan healthy meals, find recipes, and even generate shopping lists.
- **Mindfulness and Meditation:** Apps like Headspace, Calm, and Insight Timer offer guided meditations and mindfulness exercises to help manage stress and emotional eating.

When choosing an app, consider its features, user reviews, and whether it aligns with your specific needs and preferences. Many apps offer free versions with the option to upgrade to premium for additional features.

Integrating Technology into Daily Life

Integrating technology into your daily routine can significantly enhance your weight loss efforts. Here are some tips:

- **Set Reminders:** Use your phone or smartwatch to set reminders for meals, exercise, and hydration. This helps you stay on track and avoid skipping important activities.
- **Track Progress:** Regularly update your weight, measurements, and fitness progress in your chosen apps. Seeing your progress can be highly motivating.
- **Sync Devices:** If you use multiple devices (e.g., a fitness tracker and a smartphone), make sure

they are synced. This allows for seamless tracking and more accurate data.

Wearable Technology

Wearable technology, such as fitness trackers and smartwatches, can provide real-time feedback on your physical activity, sleep patterns, and even heart rate. Popular options include Fitbit, Apple Watch, Garmin, and Polar. These devices can help you:

- **Monitor Activity Levels:** Track steps, distance, and calories burned.
- **Set and Achieve Goals:** Set daily or weekly fitness goals and receive notifications and encouragement.
- **Analyze Sleep Patterns:** Understand your sleep cycles and identify areas for improvement.
- **Stay Motivated:** Receive reminders to move, notifications for reaching milestones, and motivational messages.

2. Online Communities and Support

Finding Online Communities

Online communities can provide support, motivation, and accountability on your weight loss journey. Platforms like Reddit, Facebook, and specialized forums host groups where you can share your experiences, seek advice, and celebrate successes. Some popular communities include:

- **Reddit:** Subreddits like r/loseit and r/fitness offer a wealth of information and support from fellow users.
- **Facebook Groups:** Search for weight loss groups that align with your interests and goals. Many groups are private, providing a safe space for sharing.
- **Specialized Forums:** Websites like MyFitnessPal and SparkPeople have dedicated forums for various aspects of weight loss and fitness.

Benefits of Online Support

Joining an online community can offer several benefits:

- **Accountability:** Sharing your goals and progress with others can help keep you accountable.
- **Support:** Receive encouragement and advice from people who understand your challenges.
- **Motivation:** Seeing others' success stories can inspire and motivate you to keep going.
- **Resources:** Access a wealth of information, tips, and resources shared by community members.

Engaging with the Community

To get the most out of online communities:

- **Be Active:** Regularly participate in discussions, share your progress, and offer support to others.
- **Ask Questions:** Don't hesitate to seek advice or ask for help when needed.
- **Celebrate Wins:** Share your successes, no matter how small. Celebrating milestones can boost your motivation and inspire others.

3. Tracking Your Progress Digitally

The Importance of Tracking

Tracking your progress is essential for staying motivated and making informed adjustments to your weight loss plan. Digital tools can simplify this process and provide detailed insights into your journey.

Using Digital Tools

Here are some ways to track your progress digitally:

- **Weight and Measurements:** Use a digital scale and a measuring tape to track your weight and body measurements. Input this data into a tracking app to visualize trends over time.
- **Food Diary:** Log your meals and snacks in a calorie-counting app to monitor your calorie intake and nutritional balance.

- **Exercise Log:** Record your workouts, including duration, type, and intensity. Fitness apps can track this data automatically if synced with wearable devices.
- **Health Metrics:** Some apps allow you to track additional health metrics like blood pressure, blood sugar levels, and sleep quality.

Analyzing Data

Regularly review your data to identify patterns and make necessary adjustments. For example, if you notice a plateau in your weight loss, you might analyze your calorie intake and activity levels to pinpoint potential areas for improvement.

Setting Milestones

Set short-term and long-term milestones to stay motivated. Celebrate reaching each milestone, whether it's losing a certain amount of weight, achieving a fitness goal, or sticking to your plan consistently for a set period.

4. Staying Informed with the Latest Research

The Importance of Staying Informed

The field of weight loss and fitness is constantly evolving, with new research and trends emerging regularly. Staying informed can help you adopt evidence-based practices and avoid outdated or ineffective methods.

Reliable Sources of Information

Identify reliable sources of information to stay updated:

- **Scientific Journals:** Publications like The Journal of Nutrition, Obesity, and The American Journal of Clinical Nutrition provide peer-reviewed research.
- **Health Websites:** Websites like the Mayo Clinic, WebMD, and the National Institutes of Health (NIH) offer trustworthy health information.
- **Professional Organizations:** Organizations like the American Dietetic Association (ADA) and the American College of Sports Medicine (ACSM) provide guidelines and resources.

Subscribing to Newsletters and Podcasts

Subscribing to newsletters and podcasts can help you stay informed with minimal effort. Look for reputable sources that offer regular updates on weight loss, nutrition, and fitness. Examples include:

- **Newsletters:** Precision Nutrition, Healthline, and Harvard Health Publishing.
- **Podcasts:** "The Nutrition Diva's Quick and Dirty Tips," "Food Psych," and "The Model Health Show."

Critically Evaluating Information

With the abundance of information available, it's crucial to critically evaluate what you read and hear. Consider the source, check for references to scientific studies, and be wary of sensational claims. If something sounds too good to be true, it probably is.

By leveraging technology effectively, you can enhance your weight loss journey, stay motivated, and make informed decisions. From using apps and gadgets to engaging with online communities and staying updated with the latest research, technology offers a wealth of tools and resources to support your goals. Embrace these digital advancements to create a comprehensive, personalized, and sustainable approach to weight loss.

13

THE PSYCHOLOGICAL ASPECT

1. Understanding Body Image

The Concept of Body Image

Body image refers to the way individuals perceive their physical appearance and how they believe others perceive them. This perception can significantly impact self-esteem, confidence, and overall mental health. A negative body image can lead to a variety of emotional and psychological issues, including depression, anxiety, and eating disorders.

Factors Influencing Body Image

Several factors can influence body image, including:

- **Media and Social Media:** The portrayal of idealized body types in media and social media can create unrealistic standards of beauty, leading to body dissatisfaction.

- **Cultural and Societal Norms:** Different cultures and societies have varying standards of beauty, which can impact how individuals view their bodies.
- **Family and Peer Influences:** Comments and attitudes from family and peers can shape body image perceptions from a young age.
- **Personal Experiences:** Traumatic experiences, such as bullying or weight-related teasing, can negatively affect body image.

Improving Body Image

Improving body image involves changing the way you think and feel about your body. Here are some strategies to help:

- **Practice Self-Acceptance:** Embrace your body as it is and recognize that everyone has unique features. Focus on your strengths and qualities beyond physical appearance.
- **Limit Media Consumption:** Be mindful of the media you consume. Follow accounts and consume content that promotes body positivity and diversity.
- **Surround Yourself with Positive Influences:** Spend time with people who support and uplift you. Avoid those who make negative comments about your body or appearance.

- **Engage in Positive Self-Talk:** Challenge negative thoughts about your body and replace them with positive affirmations. For example, instead of thinking, "I hate my body," say, "I am grateful for what my body can do."
- **Focus on Health, Not Weight:** Shift your focus from weight loss to overall health and well-being. Celebrate your body for its strength and capabilities.

2. The Role of Therapy

Understanding the Need for Therapy

Therapy can be a valuable tool for addressing the psychological aspects of weight loss. It provides a safe and supportive space to explore underlying issues, develop coping strategies, and foster a healthier relationship with food and your body. Therapy can be particularly beneficial for individuals struggling with emotional eating, body image issues, or past traumas related to weight.

Types of Therapy

Several types of therapy can be effective for individuals on a weight loss journey:

- **Cognitive-Behavioral Therapy (CBT):** CBT helps identify and challenge negative thought patterns and behaviors related to food and body image. It focuses on developing healthier coping mechanisms and setting realistic goals.

- **Dialectical Behavior Therapy (DBT):** DBT combines CBT with mindfulness practices to help individuals manage emotions and improve self-regulation. It can be particularly helpful for emotional eating and binge eating disorders.
- **Acceptance and Commitment Therapy (ACT):** ACT encourages individuals to accept their thoughts and feelings rather than fighting them. It focuses on commitment to values-based actions, promoting a more positive relationship with food and body.
- **Mindfulness-Based Stress Reduction (MBSR):** MBSR incorporates mindfulness and meditation practices to reduce stress and improve overall well-being. It can help individuals develop a more mindful approach to eating.

Finding the Right Therapist

Finding the right therapist is crucial for effective treatment. Look for a therapist who specializes in weight-related issues and has experience with the specific type of therapy you are interested in. It's important to feel comfortable and understood by your therapist, so don't hesitate to try a few different professionals until you find the right fit.

Integrating Therapy into Your Routine

Therapy should be integrated into your routine as a regular part of your weight loss journey. Consistent sessions can help you stay on track, address emerging issues, and maintain a positive mindset. Additionally, consider incorporating group therapy or support groups, which can provide a sense of community and shared experiences.

3. Developing a Healthy Relationship with Food

Understanding Your Relationship with Food

Your relationship with food encompasses your thoughts, feelings, and behaviors around eating. A healthy relationship with food is characterized by a balanced, flexible approach to eating that allows for both nourishment and enjoyment. Conversely, an unhealthy relationship with food may involve restrictive dieting, emotional eating, or an obsession with weight and calories.

Identifying Unhealthy Patterns

To develop a healthier relationship with food, it's important to identify any unhealthy patterns. Reflect on your eating habits and consider the following questions:

- Do you often eat when you're not hungry or use food to cope with emotions?
- Do you label foods as "good" or "bad" and feel guilty after eating certain foods?

- Do you frequently skip meals or engage in restrictive dieting?
- Do you feel out of control around food or experience binge eating episodes?

Recognizing these patterns is the first step toward change.

Mindful Eating Practices

Mindful eating involves paying full attention to the eating experience, using all your senses, and acknowledging your body's hunger and fullness cues. Here are some tips for practicing mindful eating:

- **Eat Without Distractions:** Avoid eating while watching TV, working, or using your phone. Focus solely on your meal.
- **Savor Your Food:** Take the time to appreciate the flavors, textures, and aromas of your food. Eat slowly and chew thoroughly.
- **Listen to Your Body:** Pay attention to your hunger and fullness signals. Eat when you're hungry and stop when you're satisfied, not stuffed.
- **Reflect on Your Eating Experience:** After eating, take a moment to reflect on how the meal made you feel. Did you enjoy it? Did it satisfy your hunger?

Intuitive Eating

Intuitive eating is a flexible, non-diet approach that promotes a healthy relationship with food. It involves listening to your body's natural hunger and fullness cues and rejecting the diet mentality. Key principles of intuitive eating include:

- **Reject the Diet Mentality:** Let go of the idea that you need to follow strict diets to lose weight. Trust your body to guide your eating.
- **Honor Your Hunger:** Eat when you're hungry and provide your body with adequate nourishment.
- **Make Peace with Food:** Allow yourself to enjoy all foods without guilt or restriction. Recognize that no food is off-limits.
- **Challenge the Food Police:** Challenge negative thoughts and rules about food. Trust your body's signals over external diet rules.
- **Respect Your Fullness:** Pay attention to your body's signals of fullness and stop eating when you're satisfied.
- **Discover the Satisfaction Factor:** Find joy and satisfaction in eating. Choose foods that you enjoy and that nourish your body.
- **Honor Your Feelings Without Using Food:** Find alternative ways to cope with emotions instead of turning to food.

4. Overcoming Negative Self-Talk

Understanding Negative Self-Talk

Negative self-talk refers to the critical and often harmful thoughts you have about yourself. This inner dialogue can significantly impact your self-esteem, confidence, and motivation. Common examples of negative self-talk include:

- "I'm a failure."
- "I'll never be able to lose weight."
- "I'm not good enough."
- "I don't deserve to be happy."

These thoughts can create a cycle of self-sabotage and hinder your progress on your weight loss journey.

Challenging Negative Self-Talk

To overcome negative self-talk, it's essential to challenge and reframe these thoughts. Here's how to do it:

- **Identify Negative Thoughts:** Pay attention to your inner dialogue and notice when you engage in negative self-talk. Write down these thoughts to gain awareness.
- **Examine the Evidence:** Evaluate the evidence for and against your negative thoughts. Are these thoughts based on facts or assumptions? Look for instances that contradict these thoughts.
- **Reframe Your Thoughts:** Replace negative thoughts with more positive and realistic ones. For example, if you think, "I'll never lose

weight," reframe it to, "I'm making progress and learning healthier habits every day."

- **Practice Self-Compassion:** Treat yourself with kindness and understanding. Acknowledge that everyone makes mistakes and that setbacks are a normal part of any journey.

Developing Positive Self-Talk

Positive self-talk involves cultivating an encouraging and supportive inner dialogue. Here are some tips to develop positive self-talk:

- **Affirmations:** Use positive affirmations to reinforce new beliefs. Repeat statements like, "I am capable of achieving my goals," or "I deserve to be healthy and happy."
- **Celebrate Your Achievements:** Recognize and celebrate your successes, no matter how small. This practice reinforces positive behavior and boosts motivation.
- **Focus on Your Strengths:** Identify your strengths and focus on them. Remind yourself of your abilities and accomplishments regularly.
- **Practice Gratitude:** Keep a gratitude journal and write down things you are grateful for each day. This practice shifts your focus from what's lacking to what's abundant in your life.

By addressing the psychological aspects of weight loss, including body image, the role of therapy, developing a healthy relationship with food, and overcoming negative self-talk, you can create a more supportive and positive mindset. These strategies will help you build a strong foundation for lasting success on your weight loss journey. Each step you take towards improving your mental and emotional well-being will bring you closer to achieving your goals and living a healthier, happier life.

14

CUSTOMIZING YOUR PLAN

1. Assessing Your Needs

Understanding Individual Differences

No two individuals are alike, and this is especially true when it comes to weight loss. Your body, lifestyle, preferences, and challenges are unique to you, which means a one-size-fits-all approach to weight loss is unlikely to be effective. Customizing your plan involves assessing your specific needs and tailoring your strategy accordingly.

Evaluating Your Current Habits

Start by conducting an honest assessment of your current habits. Keep a detailed food and activity diary for a week, noting everything you eat, drink, and do. Pay attention to:

- **Eating Patterns:** When do you eat? How often do you snack? Do you eat out of boredom or stress?
- **Food Choices:** What types of foods are you consuming? Are they nutrient-dense or calorie-dense?
- **Physical Activity:** How much physical activity do you get? What types of exercises do you enjoy?
- **Sleep Patterns:** How much sleep are you getting? Is it restful?
- **Stress Levels:** How do you cope with stress? Are there any particular stressors affecting your eating habits?

Analyzing this information can help you identify areas that need improvement and opportunities for change.

Setting Personalized Goals

Based on your self-assessment, set personalized goals that address your specific needs. For example:

- **If you find that you snack frequently out of boredom, set a goal to find alternative activities to engage in during those times.**
- **If your diet lacks fruits and vegetables, aim to incorporate a serving into each meal.**
- **If you are not getting enough exercise, set a goal to walk for 30 minutes each day.**

Ensure that these goals are realistic and tailored to your lifestyle.

2. Creating a Personalized Strategy

Designing Your Meal Plan

Creating a meal plan that suits your tastes and nutritional needs is crucial. Consider the following when designing your plan:

- **Nutrient Balance:** Ensure your meals include a balance of protein, healthy fats, and carbohydrates. Focus on whole, unprocessed foods.
- **Portion Control:** Be mindful of portion sizes to avoid overeating. Using smaller plates and measuring servings can help.
- **Variety:** Incorporate a variety of foods to prevent boredom and ensure you're getting a range of nutrients.
- **Flexibility:** Allow for flexibility in your meal plan to accommodate special occasions or cravings. A rigid plan can lead to frustration and potential relapse.

Incorporating Enjoyable Activities

Exercise should be enjoyable and sustainable. Find activities that you look forward to rather than see as a chore. Consider:

- **Mixing It Up:** Include a mix of cardio, strength training, and flexibility exercises.
- **Social Activities:** Join a sports team, exercise class, or find a workout buddy to make physical activity more enjoyable.
- **Hobbies:** Incorporate active hobbies like dancing, hiking, or gardening.

Addressing Specific Challenges

Your weight loss journey may come with unique challenges that require specific strategies. For example:

- **Medical Conditions:** If you have a medical condition such as diabetes or hypothyroidism, work with your healthcare provider to tailor your plan.
- **Time Constraints:** If you have a busy schedule, look for quick and easy meal options and incorporate short, effective workouts.
- **Family Dynamics:** If family meals are a challenge, find healthy recipes that everyone enjoys and involve family members in meal preparation.

3. Adapting as You Progress

Regular Monitoring and Adjustment

As you progress, regularly monitor your results and adjust your plan as needed. Track your weight, measurements, and other indicators of progress, such as energy levels and mood. Reflect on:

- **What's Working:** Identify strategies that are effective and enjoyable.
- **What's Not Working:** Pinpoint areas where you're struggling and need to make changes.

Make adjustments to your diet, exercise routine, and other habits based on this feedback.

Staying Flexible

Flexibility is crucial for long-term success. Life is unpredictable, and your weight loss plan should be adaptable to different circumstances. For instance:

- **Travel:** Learn how to make healthy choices when eating out or traveling.
- **Special Occasions:** Find ways to enjoy celebrations without derailing your progress.
- **Plateaus:** If you hit a plateau, experiment with different strategies, such as changing your workout routine or adjusting your calorie intake.

Remember, flexibility doesn't mean abandoning your goals but rather finding ways to stay on track in various situations.

Seeking Feedback and Support

Regularly seek feedback and support from others. This could be a weight loss group, a personal trainer, a dietitian, or supportive friends and family. Sharing your journey with others can provide motivation, accountability, and new insights.

4. Maintaining Flexibility

Long-Term Sustainability

For weight loss to be sustainable, it must fit into your lifestyle long-term. This means avoiding extreme diets or exercise routines that are not maintainable. Instead, focus on making gradual, sustainable changes that you can stick with for life.

Building a Supportive Environment

Create an environment that supports your weight loss goals. This might include:

- **Healthy Home:** Keep your home stocked with healthy foods and free from high-calorie temptations.
- **Supportive Social Circle:** Surround yourself with people who support your goals and encourage healthy habits.
- **Healthy Habits:** Develop habits that make healthy choices easier, such as meal prepping, scheduling regular exercise, and practicing mindfulness.

Continuing Education and Adaptation

Stay informed about nutrition, fitness, and health. Science and recommendations evolve, and staying educated can help you make informed decisions. Adapt your plan as new information becomes available and as your body and lifestyle change over time.

Celebrating Progress and Adjusting Goals

Regularly celebrate your progress and set new goals. Acknowledge your achievements, no matter how small, and use them as motivation to keep going. As you reach your initial goals, set new ones to continue challenging yourself and maintaining your progress.

Customizing your weight loss plan ensures that it fits your unique needs and lifestyle, making it more likely to be effective and sustainable. By assessing your needs, creating a personalized strategy, adapting as you progress, and maintaining flexibility, you can develop a plan that works for you in the long term. This approach not only enhances your chances of success but also helps you build a healthier, happier lifestyle.

15

THE LONG-TERM PERSPECTIVE

I. Preparing for Maintenance

Understanding the Maintenance Phase

The maintenance phase of weight loss is crucial for sustaining your achievements and avoiding the common pitfall of regaining lost weight. It's not just about reaching your goal but about maintaining a healthy lifestyle indefinitely. This phase involves shifting focus from weight loss to weight maintenance, which requires a balance of continued healthy habits, ongoing self-monitoring, and adaptability to new life circumstances.

Establishing Long-Term Habits

During the weight loss phase, you developed various habits and routines that contributed to your success. These habits need to be continued and adapted for long-term maintenance. Focus on the following:

- **Consistent Eating Patterns:** Maintain a balanced diet that includes a variety of foods. Avoid drastic diets and instead aim for sustainability.
- **Regular Physical Activity:** Continue with an exercise routine that you enjoy and can sustain. Incorporate a mix of cardiovascular exercises, strength training, and flexibility exercises.
- **Hydration and Sleep:** Ensure you stay hydrated and get sufficient sleep, as both are crucial for overall health and weight maintenance.

Self-Monitoring and Accountability

Regular self-monitoring can help you stay on track. This could involve:

- **Weighing Yourself:** Regularly weigh yourself, but not obsessively. Once a week can be a good frequency.
- **Keeping a Food Diary:** Continue tracking what you eat to remain mindful of your food choices.
- **Monitoring Physical Activity:** Use apps or journals to keep track of your exercise routines and progress.

Accountability can also play a significant role in maintenance. Stay connected with support groups, friends, or a coach who can help keep you motivated and accountable.

Adapting to New Challenges

Life is dynamic, and new challenges will arise. Whether it's a change in job, moving to a new place, or personal events, these changes can impact your routine. Prepare to adapt your strategies to fit new circumstances while maintaining your healthy habits. Flexibility and resilience are key.

2. Preventing Weight Regain

Understanding Why Weight Regain Happens

Weight regain is common due to several factors, including metabolic adaptation, hormonal changes, and reverting to old habits. Understanding these factors can help you devise strategies to prevent them.

- **Metabolic Adaptation:** As you lose weight, your metabolism slows down. It's important to adjust your caloric intake and activity level to match your new metabolic rate.
- **Hormonal Changes:** Hormones like ghrelin (hunger hormone) can increase, making you feel hungrier. Manage these changes by focusing on high-fiber and high-protein foods that promote satiety.
- **Behavioral Patterns:** Falling back into old eating and activity habits can lead to weight regain. Stay vigilant and proactive in

maintaining the healthy habits you've developed.

Strategies to Prevent Weight Regain

- **Consistent Routine:** Stick to the routine that helped you lose weight. Regular meals, exercise, and sleep should continue to be priorities.
- **Mindful Eating:** Pay attention to hunger and fullness cues. Avoid emotional eating and practice mindful eating techniques.
- **Continued Goal Setting:** Set new goals to keep yourself motivated. These could be fitness-related, like running a 5k, or health-related, like improving your cholesterol levels.
- **Regular Check-ins:** Periodically assess your progress and make necessary adjustments. This can involve tweaking your diet, modifying your exercise routine, or seeking additional support.

3. Continuing Healthy Habits

Building a Healthy Environment

Your environment plays a significant role in your ability to maintain weight loss. Create a supportive environment by:

- **Stocking Healthy Foods:** Keep your kitchen stocked with nutritious options and limit processed foods.
- **Creating Exercise Opportunities:** Make physical activity a natural part of your environment. Set up a home gym, take regular walks, or find local fitness classes.
- **Limiting Temptations:** Identify and minimize environmental triggers that lead to unhealthy eating or inactivity.

Maintaining Social Support

Surround yourself with people who support your healthy lifestyle. This could be friends, family, or a community of like-minded individuals. Engage in social activities that align with your goals, such as group workouts or healthy cooking classes.

Continual Learning and Adaptation

Stay informed about nutrition and fitness trends, but be critical of fad diets and unproven methods. Continue learning about healthy living through reputable sources. Adapt your strategies as you learn more about what works best for your body and lifestyle.

4. Setting New Goals

The Importance of New Goals

Setting new goals helps keep you motivated and engaged in your journey. These goals don't necessarily have to be related to weight but can encompass overall health and well-being.

- **Fitness Goals:** Aim to improve your physical fitness, whether it's through strength, flexibility, endurance, or a new sport.
- **Health Metrics:** Focus on improving or maintaining other health metrics, such as blood pressure, cholesterol levels, or blood sugar levels.
- **Personal Development:** Set goals related to personal growth, such as learning a new skill, developing a hobby, or achieving work-life balance.

SMART Goals for Long-Term Success

Continue using the SMART framework to set specific, measurable, achievable, relevant, and time-bound goals. This structured approach ensures clarity and feasibility.

Celebrating Milestones

Acknowledge and celebrate your achievements, both big and small. This could involve rewarding yourself with something non-food-related, like a new fitness gadget, a spa day, or a mini-vacation. Celebrating milestones helps reinforce positive behavior and keeps you motivated.

Reflecting on Your Journey

Take time to reflect on your journey. Recognize how far you've come, the challenges you've overcome, and the progress you've made. Reflecting on your achievements can boost your confidence and commitment to maintaining your healthy lifestyle.

By focusing on long-term strategies for maintenance, preventing weight regain, continuing healthy habits, and setting new goals, you ensure that your weight loss journey translates into a lifelong commitment to health and well-being. Each step in this chapter is designed to help you build a sustainable lifestyle that supports your goals and enhances your quality of life.

16

INSPIRING SUCCESS STORIES

1. Real-Life Transformations

Understanding the Power of Success Stories

Success stories are a powerful motivational tool. They provide tangible evidence that weight loss is achievable, offering inspiration and hope to those who may feel their goals are out of reach. Real-life transformations show that, regardless of the starting point, perseverance and dedication can lead to remarkable results.

Success Story 1: Jane's Journey

Background: Jane, a 45-year-old mother of three, had struggled with her weight for most of her adult life. After multiple failed attempts to lose weight through fad diets, she felt discouraged and resigned to being overweight.

Approach: Jane decided to take a different approach by focusing on sustainable lifestyle changes. She started by setting small, manageable goals, such as walking for 20 minutes a day and incorporating more vegetables into her diet. Jane also sought support from a local weight loss group, which provided her with accountability and encouragement.

Transformation: Over the course of a year, Jane lost 50 pounds. She attributes her success to the slow and steady approach, the support of her weight loss group, and her newfound love for cooking healthy meals. Jane now enjoys an active lifestyle and has maintained her weight loss for over two years.

Key Takeaway: Small, sustainable changes and a strong support system can lead to long-term success.

Success Story 2: Mark's Breakthrough

Background: Mark, a 32-year-old office worker, had been overweight since his teenage years. He had a sedentary job and struggled with emotional eating, using food as a way to cope with stress and anxiety.

Approach: Mark decided to address his weight issues by focusing on both his physical and emotional health. He began seeing a therapist to work on his emotional eating and stress management. Simultaneously, he started a beginner-friendly exercise routine and made gradual dietary changes, such as reducing his intake of sugary drinks.

Transformation: In 18 months, Mark lost 60 pounds. He now practices mindfulness and meditation to manage stress and has developed a consistent exercise routine that includes running and weight training. Mark feels more energetic and confident, and his mental health has significantly improved.

Key Takeaway: Addressing emotional health and building a balanced routine are crucial for successful weight loss.

Success Story 3: Emily's Lifestyle Change

Background: Emily, a 28-year-old nurse, found herself gaining weight due to irregular work hours and unhealthy eating habits. She felt tired and unhappy with her appearance, but her busy schedule made it challenging to prioritize her health.

Approach: Emily started by making small changes that fit into her hectic lifestyle. She began meal prepping on her days off, focusing on nutritious and convenient meals. Emily also started incorporating short, high-intensity interval training (HIIT) workouts into her routine, which she could do at home.

Transformation: Emily lost 40 pounds over the course of a year. She now has more energy to perform her demanding job and feels more confident in her body. The key to her success was finding a balance that worked with her schedule and staying consistent with her healthy habits.

Key Takeaway: Adapting healthy habits to fit a busy lifestyle can lead to significant weight loss success.

2. Learning from Others' Journeys

Common Themes and Strategies

By examining these success stories, several common themes and strategies emerge that can be applied to your own weight loss journey:

- **Setting Realistic Goals:** Each individual set achievable goals that allowed for steady progress.
- **Consistency:** Sustainable, long-term changes were prioritized over quick fixes.
- **Support Systems:** Whether through therapy, support groups, or friends and family, having a support system was crucial.
- **Mindfulness and Self-Compassion:** Addressing emotional health and practicing self-compassion helped manage stress and prevent setbacks.
- **Adapting to Lifestyle:** Successful individuals found ways to incorporate healthy habits into their existing routines, making changes that were practical and sustainable.

Implementing These Strategies

To implement these strategies in your own journey, start by setting realistic and specific goals. Identify areas where you can make gradual changes, such as improving your diet or increasing your physical activity. Seek out support, whether from a weight loss group, a therapist, or supportive friends and family. Practice mindfulness and self-compassion to manage stress and stay motivated. Finally, find ways to adapt healthy habits to fit your lifestyle, ensuring that changes are sustainable.

3. Common Success Strategies

Strategy 1: Incremental Changes

Many success stories highlight the importance of incremental changes. Instead of overhauling their entire lifestyle overnight, successful individuals made small, manageable changes that added up over time. This approach prevents overwhelm and makes it easier to stick with new habits.

How to Apply: Start by identifying one or two small changes you can make. This might include drinking more water, adding an extra serving of vegetables to your meals, or taking a short walk each day. Once these changes become routine, gradually add more.

Strategy 2: Building a Support Network

Having a strong support network is a common factor in many weight loss success stories. Support can come from various sources, including friends, family, weight loss groups, or online communities. These networks provide encouragement, accountability, and a sense of camaraderie.

How to Apply: Reach out to friends or family members who are supportive of your goals. Consider joining a weight loss group or finding an online community where you can share your journey and gain support from others facing similar challenges.

Strategy 3: Embracing a Balanced Approach

A balanced approach to weight loss focuses on creating a healthy relationship with food and exercise, rather than following restrictive diets or extreme workout regimens. Successful individuals often emphasize the importance of moderation and enjoying a variety of foods.

How to Apply: Aim for balance in your diet by including a variety of nutrient-dense foods. Allow yourself occasional treats without guilt. Find physical activities you enjoy and incorporate them into your routine, ensuring that exercise feels like a positive and rewarding part of your life.

Strategy 4: Tracking Progress

Tracking progress helps maintain motivation and provides valuable insights into what's working and what needs adjustment. Many successful individuals keep track of their food intake, physical activity, and weight to monitor their progress.

How to Apply: Use a journal, app, or spreadsheet to track your food, exercise, and weight. Review your entries regularly to identify patterns and make necessary adjustments. Celebrate your progress, no matter how small, to stay motivated.

Strategy 5: Prioritizing Mental Health

Addressing mental health is a crucial aspect of successful weight loss. Many individuals find that managing stress, emotional eating, and self-esteem issues is key to their success. Practices such as mindfulness, meditation, and therapy can be incredibly beneficial.

How to Apply: Incorporate mindfulness or meditation into your daily routine. Consider seeking therapy if you struggle with emotional eating or self-esteem issues. Prioritize self-care and stress management to support your mental well-being.

4. Staying Inspired

Finding Ongoing Inspiration

Staying inspired throughout your weight loss journey can be challenging, especially during difficult times. Finding ongoing inspiration is essential to keep you motivated and focused on your goals.

- **Follow Inspirational Accounts:** Social media can be a great source of inspiration. Follow accounts that share positive and motivational content related to weight loss and healthy living.
- **Read Success Stories:** Regularly read or watch success stories to remind yourself of

what's possible. Seeing others achieve their goals can reignite your motivation and determination.

- **Set Short-Term Goals:** In addition to your long-term goals, set short-term goals that provide frequent opportunities for success and celebration. These can keep you engaged and motivated.
- **Create a Vision Board:** A vision board can help you visualize your goals and stay focused on your desired outcomes. Include images, quotes, and affirmations that inspire you.

Staying Motivated During Plateaus

Weight loss plateaus are a common and often frustrating part of the journey. Staying motivated during these times requires patience and perseverance.

- **Reassess Your Plan:** Use plateaus as an opportunity to reassess your plan. Are there adjustments you can make to your diet or exercise routine?
- **Focus on Non-Scale Victories:** Celebrate non-scale victories, such as improved fitness levels, better mood, or increased energy. These are important indicators of progress.
- **Stay Positive:** Maintain a positive mindset and remind yourself that plateaus are temporary. Stay committed to your goals and trust that progress will resume.

Connecting with a Community

Being part of a community can provide ongoing support and inspiration. Whether online or in-person, communities offer a space to share experiences, challenges, and successes.

- **Join Support Groups:** Look for local or online support groups focused on weight loss and healthy living. These groups can provide accountability, encouragement, and practical advice.
- **Participate in Challenges:** Many communities organize weight loss challenges or fitness competitions. Participating in these can add a fun and competitive element to your journey.
- **Share Your Story:** Consider sharing your own journey within your community. Not only can this inspire others, but it can also reinforce your commitment to your goals.

By drawing inspiration from real-life success stories and learning from the common strategies employed by those who have achieved their weight loss goals, you can find motivation and practical advice for your own journey. Remember, weight loss is not just about the physical transformation but also about improving your overall well-being and adopting a healthier lifestyle.

Stay inspired, stay committed, and trust in your ability to achieve your goals.

17

———————

THE ROLE OF PROFESSIONAL HELP

1. Working with a Nutritionist

The Benefits of Professional Guidance

Navigating the complexities of nutrition can be daunting, especially when trying to lose weight. A nutritionist provides personalized guidance tailored to your specific needs and goals. They can help you understand your dietary needs, create a balanced meal plan, and provide accountability.

Finding the Right Nutritionist

When looking for a nutritionist, it's essential to find someone who is qualified and whose approach aligns with your goals. Look for registered dietitians (RD) or licensed nutritionists who have the appropriate certifications and experience. Ask for recommendations, read reviews, and schedule an initial consultation to ensure a good fit.

What to Expect in Your First Appointment

During your first appointment, the nutritionist will typically conduct a thorough assessment, including your medical history, current diet, lifestyle, and weight loss goals. They will use this information to create a personalized plan that may include specific dietary recommendations, meal planning tips, and strategies to overcome any challenges you might face.

Creating a Sustainable Eating Plan

A key aspect of working with a nutritionist is developing a sustainable eating plan that you can stick to long-term. This plan should balance your nutritional needs with your personal preferences and lifestyle. The nutritionist will help you make gradual, manageable changes to your diet that promote weight loss and overall health without feeling restrictive.

2. The Benefits of a Personal Trainer

Personalized Exercise Plans

Just as a nutritionist can tailor a meal plan to your needs, a personal trainer can create a personalized exercise program that suits your fitness level, preferences, and goals. They can introduce you to new exercises, ensure you are using proper form to prevent injuries, and progressively increase the intensity of your workouts as you become more fit.

Motivation and Accountability

One of the significant advantages of working with a personal trainer is the added motivation and accountability. Scheduled sessions provide structure and commitment, making it harder to skip workouts. A trainer can also help you set realistic fitness goals and celebrate your progress, keeping you motivated throughout your journey.

Finding the Right Trainer

Choosing the right personal trainer is crucial. Look for certified trainers with experience and positive reviews. It's also essential to find someone whose training style matches your preferences. Some people thrive with a more intense, military-style approach, while others may prefer a more supportive and gentle style.

In-Person vs. Online Training

With the rise of technology, many trainers offer online sessions, which can be a flexible and cost-effective option. Online training allows you to work out from home with professional guidance, while in-person training provides hands-on support and direct interaction. Consider your needs and preferences when deciding between the two.

3. Seeking Psychological Support

Understanding the Psychological Aspects of Weight Loss

Weight loss is not just a physical challenge but a psychological one as well. Emotional eating, stress, and negative self-image are common barriers that can impede progress. Seeking psychological support can help address these issues, providing tools and strategies to overcome them.

Types of Psychological Support

- **Therapists and Counselors:** These professionals can help you explore the emotional and mental factors contributing to weight gain. Cognitive-behavioral therapy (CBT) is particularly effective for changing unhealthy behaviors and thought patterns.
- **Support Groups:** Joining a weight loss support group can provide a sense of community and shared experience. These groups offer emotional support, practical tips, and encouragement from others who are on a similar journey.
- **Mindfulness and Stress Reduction Programs:** Programs focused on mindfulness and stress reduction, such as mindfulness-based stress reduction (MBSR), can help you manage stress and emotional eating.

Finding the Right Support

When seeking psychological support, it's important to find a professional who specializes in weight management and has experience with the unique challenges you face. Recommendations from your primary care physician, nutritionist, or personal trainer can be valuable.

Integrating Psychological Strategies

Incorporating psychological strategies into your weight loss plan can enhance your overall success. Techniques such as mindfulness meditation, journaling, and relaxation exercises can help you stay focused, manage stress, and maintain a positive mindset.

4. Using Medical Interventions Wisely

Understanding Medical Options

For some individuals, medical interventions may be necessary to achieve significant weight loss. These interventions should be considered carefully and discussed with your healthcare provider. Options include prescription medications, weight loss surgery, and medically supervised weight loss programs.

Prescription Medications

There are several medications available that can aid in weight loss by suppressing appetite, reducing fat absorption, or increasing feelings of fullness. These medications are typically prescribed for individuals with a BMI over 30 or those with weight-related health issues. It's important to discuss the potential benefits and side effects with your doctor.

Weight Loss Surgery

Weight loss surgery, such as gastric bypass, gastric sleeve, or lap band surgery, may be an option for individuals with severe obesity who have not had success with other weight loss methods. These procedures can result in significant weight loss and improvement in obesity-related conditions but also come with risks and require lifelong dietary changes and monitoring.

Medically Supervised Weight Loss Programs

These programs often combine medical, nutritional, and psychological support to help you lose weight safely and effectively. They may include meal replacements, low-calorie diets, and regular monitoring by healthcare professionals. Such programs are typically recommended for those with significant weight to lose or those who have struggled with traditional weight loss methods.

Evaluating the Risks and Benefits

Before considering any medical intervention, it's crucial to thoroughly evaluate the risks and benefits. Discuss your options with your healthcare provider, and consider seeking a second opinion if necessary. Ensure that you understand the commitment required and the potential impact on your life.

Working with a Nutritionist

Working with a nutritionist can provide the guidance and support needed to make lasting dietary changes. Here's how to maximize the benefits of this professional relationship:

Creating a Tailored Meal Plan

A nutritionist will work with you to create a meal plan that fits your lifestyle, preferences, and nutritional needs. This plan will likely include:

- **Balanced Meals:** Emphasizing whole foods, lean proteins, healthy fats, and complex carbohydrates.
- **Portion Control:** Learning to recognize appropriate portion sizes to avoid overeating.
- **Meal Timing:** Structuring meals and snacks to maintain energy levels and prevent hunger.
- **Hydration:** Ensuring adequate fluid intake throughout the day.

Addressing Dietary Challenges

A nutritionist can help you overcome common dietary challenges, such as:

- **Emotional Eating:** Identifying triggers and developing healthier coping mechanisms.
- **Food Intolerances/Allergies:** Creating a meal plan that avoids problematic foods while ensuring nutritional balance.

- **Busy Lifestyle:** Finding quick and healthy
  meal options for on-the-go eating.

Ongoing Support and Accountability

Regular follow-up appointments with your nutritionist can provide accountability and support. They can help you track your progress, adjust your meal plan as needed, and address any challenges that arise. This ongoing support is crucial for maintaining motivation and ensuring long-term success.

The Benefits of a Personal Trainer

Engaging a personal trainer can significantly enhance your fitness journey. Here's how to make the most of this professional relationship:

Personalized Exercise Program

A personal trainer will design an exercise program tailored to your fitness level, goals, and preferences. This program will likely include:

- **Cardiovascular Exercise:** Activities that
  increase heart rate and improve
  cardiovascular health.
- **Strength Training:** Exercises that build
  muscle, improve metabolism, and enhance
  overall strength.
- **Flexibility and Mobility:** Stretching and
  mobility exercises to prevent injury and

improve movement.

- **Progressive Overload:** Gradually increasing the intensity of your workouts to continually challenge your body and prevent plateaus.

Motivation and Accountability

A personal trainer provides motivation and accountability, helping you stay committed to your fitness goals. They can:

- **Set Realistic Goals:** Helping you set achievable fitness goals and creating a plan to reach them.
- **Monitor Progress:** Tracking your progress and adjusting your program as needed.
- **Provide Encouragement:** Offering support and encouragement to keep you motivated.

Preventing Injury

Proper form and technique are crucial to preventing injuries. A personal trainer will:

- **Teach Proper Technique:** Ensuring you perform exercises correctly to avoid injury.
- **Monitor Your Form:** Providing real-time feedback to correct any mistakes.
- **Adapt Exercises:** Modifying exercises to suit your abilities and limitations.

Building Confidence

Working with a personal trainer can boost your confidence in your abilities. As you progress, you'll gain a sense of accomplishment and self-assurance in your physical capabilities.

Seeking Psychological Support

Addressing the psychological aspects of weight loss is critical for long-term success. Here's how to effectively integrate psychological support into your journey:

Understanding Emotional Eating

Emotional eating is a common barrier to weight loss. It involves using food to cope with emotions such as stress, boredom, or sadness. A therapist or counselor can help you:

- **Identify Triggers:** Recognizing the emotions or situations that lead to overeating.
- **Develop Coping Strategies:** Creating healthier ways to manage emotions, such as exercise, journaling, or mindfulness.
- **Build Emotional Awareness:** Increasing your awareness of your emotional state and its impact on your eating habits.

Cognitive-Behavioral Therapy (CBT)

CBT is an effective approach for addressing negative thought patterns and behaviors related to weight loss. A therapist can help you:

- **Challenge Negative Thoughts:** Identifying and challenging unhelpful thoughts that contribute to unhealthy eating behaviors.
- **Develop Positive Behaviors:** Creating new, healthy habits to replace old, detrimental ones.
- **Set Realistic Goals:** Establishing achievable goals and creating a plan to reach them.

Support Groups

Joining a weight loss support group can provide a sense of community and shared experience. These groups offer:

- **Emotional Support:** Connecting with others who understand your struggles and can offer empathy and encouragement.
- **Practical Tips:** Sharing strategies and tips for overcoming common challenges.
- **Accountability:** Providing a sense of accountability and motivation to stay on track.

Mindfulness and Stress Reduction

Mindfulness and stress reduction techniques can help you manage stress and emotional eating. Practices such as mindfulness meditation, deep breathing exercises, and yoga can:

- **Reduce Stress:** Lowering stress levels and reducing the likelihood of stress-related eating.

- **Increase Awareness:** Enhancing your awareness of your body and mind, helping you make more conscious choices about food.
- **Promote Relaxation:** Encouraging relaxation and overall well-being.

Using Medical Interventions Wisely

Medical interventions can be a valuable tool for some individuals in their weight loss journey. Here's how to approach these options wisely:

Prescription Medications

Prescription medications can aid in weight loss by suppressing appetite, reducing fat absorption, or increasing feelings of fullness. It's essential to:

- **Consult Your Doctor:** Discuss the potential benefits and risks with your healthcare provider.
- **Follow Instructions:** Use the medication as prescribed and follow your doctor's recommendations.
- **Monitor Progress:** Regularly monitor your progress and report any side effects to your doctor.

Weight Loss Surgery

Weight loss surgery may be an option for individuals with severe obesity who have not had success with other methods. Types of surgery include:

- **Gastric Bypass:** Reduces the size of the stomach and reroutes the digestive system.
- **Gastric Sleeve:** Removes a portion of the stomach to reduce its size.
- **Lap Band:** Places a band around the stomach to limit food intake.

Considerations for weight loss surgery include:

- **Eligibility:** Typically recommended for individuals with a BMI over 40 or those with obesity-related health conditions.
- **Risks and Benefits:** Understanding the potential risks and benefits, including the need for lifelong dietary changes and monitoring.
- **Commitment:** Recognizing the commitment required for post-surgery lifestyle changes.

Medically Supervised Weight Loss Programs

These programs offer comprehensive support, including medical, nutritional, and psychological guidance. They may include:

- **Meal Replacements:** Using meal replacements to control calorie intake.

- **Low-Calorie Diets:** Following a structured low-calorie diet plan.
- **Regular Monitoring:** Regular check-ins with healthcare professionals to monitor progress and make adjustments.

Evaluating Options

Before considering any medical intervention, it's essential to:

- **Research Thoroughly:** Understand the potential benefits, risks, and requirements of each option.
- **Consult Healthcare Providers:** Discuss your options with your primary care physician and specialists.
- **Seek a Second Opinion:** Consider seeking a second opinion to ensure you make an informed decision.

By incorporating professional help into your weight loss journey, you can benefit from personalized guidance, support, and expertise. Whether working with a nutritionist, personal trainer, therapist, or exploring medical interventions, these resources can provide the tools and strategies needed to achieve and maintain your weight loss goals.

18

ADDRESSING COMMON PITFALLS

1. Identifying Potential Roadblocks

Understanding Common Pitfalls

Despite the best intentions and carefully crafted plans, many people encounter obstacles on their weight loss journey. These pitfalls can vary widely, from physical challenges and emotional hurdles to environmental and social influences. Identifying these potential roadblocks early can help you prepare strategies to overcome them. Common pitfalls include:

- **Plateaus:** Hitting a weight loss plateau where progress stalls despite ongoing efforts.
- **Emotional Eating:** Using food as a coping mechanism for stress, boredom, or other emotions.
- **Lack of Time:** Struggling to find time for meal preparation and exercise.

- **Social Pressures:** Facing pressure to indulge in unhealthy foods at social gatherings.
- **Inconsistent Motivation:** Losing motivation and falling back into old habits.

Personalizing Your Pitfall Plan

Everyone's journey is unique, and so are the obstacles they face. Reflect on your past experiences and identify specific challenges that have hindered your progress. Create a personalized list of potential pitfalls and think about what triggers these challenges. Understanding your personal roadblocks is the first step toward developing effective strategies to address them.

2. Strategies to Overcome Obstacles

Dealing with Plateaus

Weight loss plateaus are a common and frustrating part of the journey. They occur when your body adapts to your current routine, causing progress to stall. Here are some strategies to overcome plateaus:

- **Reevaluate Your Diet:** Make sure your calorie intake is appropriate for your current weight and activity level. Consider reducing portion sizes or cutting back on certain foods.
- **Increase Physical Activity:** Introduce new exercises or increase the intensity of your current workouts to challenge your body.

- **Track Your Progress:** Keep detailed records of your food intake and exercise. This can help identify patterns and areas for improvement.
- **Stay Hydrated:** Sometimes, the body retains water, which can affect weight loss. Ensure you're drinking enough water daily.

Managing Emotional Eating

Emotional eating can sabotage weight loss efforts by leading to overeating and poor food choices. To manage emotional eating:

- **Identify Triggers:** Keep a food diary to track what you eat, how much you eat, and your emotional state at the time. Look for patterns that indicate emotional triggers.
- **Find Alternatives:** Develop a list of alternative activities to cope with emotions, such as going for a walk, practicing yoga, calling a friend, or engaging in a hobby.
- **Practice Mindful Eating:** Slow down and pay attention to what you're eating. Focus on the taste, texture, and enjoyment of your food, and avoid distractions like watching TV while eating.
- **Seek Support:** Talking to a therapist or joining a support group can provide valuable tools and encouragement to overcome emotional eating.

Overcoming Lack of Time

Busy schedules can make it challenging to prioritize healthy eating and exercise. Here are some strategies to manage your time effectively:

- **Meal Prep:** Dedicate a few hours each week to prepare healthy meals and snacks. This can save time and reduce the temptation to opt for unhealthy options.
- **Exercise Efficiently:** Incorporate high-intensity interval training (HIIT) or other time-efficient workouts that provide maximum benefit in a shorter period.
- **Plan Ahead:** Schedule your workouts and meal prep sessions in advance, treating them as non-negotiable appointments.
- **Multitask:** Combine exercise with other activities, such as walking during phone calls or doing bodyweight exercises while watching TV.

Navigating Social Pressures

Social events and gatherings can present challenges to maintaining healthy habits. To navigate these situations:

- **Plan Ahead:** Eat a healthy meal or snack before attending an event to reduce the temptation to indulge.

- **Bring Healthy Options:** If possible, contribute a healthy dish to share at social gatherings.
- **Practice Portion Control:** Allow yourself to enjoy small portions of your favorite foods rather than depriving yourself, which can lead to overeating later.
- **Communicate Your Goals:** Let friends and family know about your weight loss goals and ask for their support. They may be more understanding and accommodating than you expect.

Maintaining Consistent Motivation

Maintaining motivation over the long term can be challenging, but these strategies can help:

- **Set Short-Term Goals:** Break down your overall goal into smaller, achievable milestones. Celebrate each success to stay motivated.
- **Visualize Your Success:** Regularly remind yourself of your reasons for losing weight and visualize the benefits you'll enjoy once you reach your goals.
- **Track Your Progress:** Use a journal or app to monitor your progress. Seeing how far you've come can be incredibly motivating.
- **Stay Connected:** Join a weight loss group or find an accountability partner to share your journey and stay motivated together.

3. Staying Consistent

Building Consistency

Consistency is key to achieving long-term weight loss success. It involves sticking to your plan and making healthy choices regularly. Here's how to build and maintain consistency:

- **Create a Routine:** Establish a daily routine that includes time for meal preparation, exercise, and self-care. Having a set schedule can make it easier to stay on track.
- **Prioritize Sleep:** Ensure you're getting enough sleep each night. Lack of sleep can negatively impact your motivation and energy levels, making it harder to stay consistent.
- **Stay Flexible:** Life is unpredictable, and there will be times when you can't stick to your routine. Allow for flexibility and adapt your plan as needed without feeling guilty or discouraged.

Accountability and Support

Having a support system can significantly improve your ability to stay consistent. Consider these options:

- **Find an Accountability Partner:** Partner with a friend, family member, or coworker who shares similar goals. Check in with each other regularly to stay motivated and accountable.

- **Join a Support Group:** Participate in a weight loss support group, either in person or online. Sharing your journey with others can provide encouragement and valuable insights.
- **Hire a Coach or Trainer:** If possible, work with a professional who can offer guidance, support, and accountability.

Monitoring and Adjusting

Regularly monitor your progress and adjust your plan as needed. This includes tracking your weight, measurements, food intake, and exercise. If you notice that certain strategies aren't working, be willing to make changes. Weight loss is a dynamic process, and what works for you at one stage may need to be adjusted as you progress.

4. Learning from Setbacks

Understanding Setbacks

Setbacks are an inevitable part of any weight loss journey. They can occur due to various reasons, such as a lack of motivation, life stressors, or unforeseen events. Rather than viewing setbacks as failures, it's important to see them as opportunities to learn and grow.

Reflecting on Setbacks

When you experience a setback, take time to reflect on what happened:

- **What Triggered the Setback?** Identify the circumstances or events that led to the setback. Understanding the triggers can help you avoid similar situations in the future.
- **How Did You Respond?** Reflect on how you reacted to the setback. Did you give up entirely, or were you able to get back on track quickly?
- **What Can You Learn?** Consider what you can learn from the experience. Are there changes you can make to your plan or strategies that could prevent similar setbacks?

Developing Resilience

Resilience is the ability to bounce back from setbacks and continue moving forward. Here are some strategies to build resilience:

- **Stay Positive:** Focus on the progress you've made rather than the setback itself. Remind yourself that setbacks are temporary and do not define your overall success.
- **Practice Self-Compassion:** Be kind to yourself during setbacks. Avoid harsh self-criticism and instead offer yourself encouragement and understanding.
- **Reframe Setbacks:** View setbacks as part of the learning process. Each setback provides valuable information about what works and

what doesn't. Use this knowledge to adjust your plan and improve your approach.

- **Recommit to Your Goals:** After a setback, recommit to your goals. Review your reasons for wanting to lose weight and remind yourself of the benefits you'll gain from staying on track.

Creating a Plan for Recovery

Having a plan in place for how to recover from setbacks can make it easier to get back on track. Your recovery plan might include:

- **Taking Immediate Action:** As soon as you recognize a setback, take immediate steps to correct course. This could mean planning a healthy meal, scheduling an extra workout, or reaching out to your support network.
- **Reviewing Your Goals:** Revisit your goals and remind yourself why they're important. This can help reignite your motivation and commitment.
- **Adjusting Your Plan:** If needed, make adjustments to your plan to address the factors that contributed to the setback. This might involve changing your exercise routine, modifying your diet, or seeking additional support.

By understanding and addressing common pitfalls, you can better navigate the challenges of your weight loss journey. Identifying potential roadblocks, developing strategies to overcome them, staying consistent, and learning from setbacks are essential components of long-term success. With the right mindset and tools, you can turn obstacles into opportunities and continue progressing toward your weight loss goals.

19

CELEBRATING MILESTONES

1. Recognizing Non-Scale Victories

Understanding Non-Scale Victories (NSVs)

Weight loss is often measured by the numbers on a scale, but this is just one aspect of success. Non-scale victories (NSVs) are crucial for maintaining motivation and recognizing the broader impact of your efforts. NSVs include improvements in health, fitness, mental well-being, and quality of life. Recognizing these victories can provide a more holistic view of your progress.

Examples of Non-Scale Victories

- **Physical Changes:** Noticeable changes in how your clothes fit, increased muscle tone, and improved posture.

- **Health Improvements:** Better blood pressure, cholesterol levels, blood sugar levels, and overall physical health.
- **Increased Energy:** Feeling more energetic and less fatigued throughout the day.
- **Enhanced Fitness:** Improved stamina, strength, flexibility, and endurance.
- **Mental Well-Being:** Reduced stress, anxiety, and depression, along with increased confidence and self-esteem.
- **Lifestyle Changes:** Adopting healthier eating habits, being more active, and finding enjoyment in physical activities.

Tracking Non-Scale Victories

To ensure you recognize and celebrate these victories, keep a journal or use a tracking app to document them. Reflect on these NSVs regularly to remind yourself of the progress you've made beyond just the numbers on the scale.

2. Rewarding Your Efforts

The Importance of Rewards

Rewarding yourself for reaching milestones is essential for maintaining motivation and reinforcing positive behavior. Rewards provide a sense of accomplishment and can serve as a powerful incentive to continue working toward your goals.

Choosing Meaningful Rewards

When selecting rewards, choose those that genuinely motivate you and support your overall health and well-being. Avoid using food as a reward, as this can reinforce unhealthy eating habits. Instead, consider the following ideas:

- **Experiences:** Plan a fun outing, a day trip, or an adventure you've been looking forward to.
- **Pampering:** Treat yourself to a spa day, massage, new outfit, or other self-care activities.
- **Hobbies:** Invest in a new hobby or purchase equipment for an activity you enjoy.
- **Fitness:** Buy new workout gear, sign up for a fitness class, or get a gym membership.

Creating a Reward System

Develop a reward system that aligns with your goals and milestones. For example, set small rewards for short-term goals and larger rewards for long-term achievements. This approach ensures that you have regular incentives to stay on track.

3. Reflecting on Your Journey

The Power of Reflection

Reflection is a powerful tool for personal growth and continuous improvement. By taking the time to reflect on your weight loss journey, you can gain valuable insights, recognize patterns, and identify areas for further development.

Journaling Your Progress

Keeping a journal throughout your journey allows you to document your thoughts, feelings, and experiences. Reflect on your successes, challenges, and lessons learned. Consider these prompts:

- **What were the key factors that contributed to my success?**
- **What challenges did I face, and how did I overcome them?**
- **How has my mindset changed since I started this journey?**
- **What non-scale victories have I experienced?**
- **How do I feel about my progress, and what are my next steps?**

Learning from Setbacks

Setbacks are an inevitable part of any journey. Reflecting on them allows you to learn and grow. Ask yourself:

- **What triggered this setback?**
- **What could I have done differently?**
- **How can I prevent similar setbacks in the future?**

By analyzing setbacks and extracting lessons from them, you can build resilience and improve your strategies moving forward.

4. Planning for the Future

Setting New Goals

As you achieve your weight loss milestones, it's important to set new goals to maintain momentum and continue your progress. These goals can be related to further weight loss, fitness achievements, personal development, or other areas of your life.

- **Fitness Goals:** Aim for new physical challenges, such as running a race, hiking a difficult trail, or mastering a new sport.
- **Health Goals:** Focus on maintaining or improving your health metrics, such as blood pressure, cholesterol, or overall wellness.
- **Personal Growth:** Set goals related to personal development, such as learning a new skill, pursuing a hobby, or enhancing your mental well-being.

Developing a Maintenance Plan

Once you've reached your weight loss goals, developing a maintenance plan is crucial to ensure long-term success. This plan should include:

- **Sustainable Eating Habits:** Continue with a balanced, nutritious diet that you can maintain long-term.
- **Regular Physical Activity:** Keep up with a consistent exercise routine that you enjoy.

- **Ongoing Monitoring:** Regularly check in on your progress and make adjustments as needed.
- **Support System:** Maintain connections with supportive friends, family, or groups.

Staying Motivated

Staying motivated after reaching your goals can be challenging. To keep your motivation high:

- **Celebrate Your Successes:** Regularly acknowledge and celebrate your achievements, both big and small.
- **Stay Inspired:** Continue to seek out inspiration through success stories, motivational content, or new challenges.
- **Find Joy in the Journey:** Focus on enjoying the process of maintaining a healthy lifestyle rather than just the outcomes.

By recognizing and celebrating your milestones, you reinforce positive behaviors and maintain motivation on your weight loss journey. Tracking non-scale victories, rewarding your efforts, reflecting on your progress, and planning for the future are essential components of long-term success. Embrace each step of your journey and continue to set new goals that inspire and challenge you.

20

EMBRACING A NEW LIFESTYLE

1. Making Permanent Changes

Understanding the Need for Permanent Changes

Achieving your weight loss goal is a significant milestone, but maintaining your new weight and lifestyle is an ongoing journey. To avoid falling back into old habits, it's essential to make permanent changes that support a healthy lifestyle. This means adopting behaviors that become part of your daily routine and are sustainable in the long run.

Identifying Sustainable Habits

Sustainable habits are those that you can maintain comfortably over time. They should fit into your lifestyle without feeling like a burden. Examples of sustainable habits include:

- **Balanced Eating:** Prioritizing whole foods, such as fruits, vegetables, lean proteins, and whole grains, while allowing occasional treats in moderation.
- **Regular Physical Activity:** Incorporating activities you enjoy, whether it's walking, dancing, cycling, or yoga, into your routine.
- **Mindful Eating:** Paying attention to hunger and fullness cues, eating slowly, and savoring your food.
- **Hydration:** Drinking plenty of water throughout the day to stay hydrated.
- **Sleep Hygiene:** Maintaining a regular sleep schedule and creating a restful environment for quality sleep.

Building a New Routine

Creating a new routine involves integrating your sustainable habits into your daily life. Start by setting a schedule that includes time for meal preparation, exercise, and relaxation. Use tools like calendars, planners, or apps to help you stay organized and committed.

Consider the following steps to build your new routine:

- **Morning Ritual:** Start your day with a healthy breakfast, a glass of water, and a few minutes of stretching or meditation.

- **Meal Planning:** Plan your meals and snacks for the week to ensure you have healthy options readily available.
- **Exercise Schedule:** Set specific times for physical activity, whether it's a morning jog, a lunchtime walk, or an evening yoga session.
- **Evening Routine:** Wind down with a relaxing activity like reading, journaling, or a warm bath to prepare for a restful night's sleep.

Adapting to Life Changes

Life is dynamic, and your routine may need to adapt to changes such as a new job, moving to a different location, or changes in family responsibilities. Stay flexible and open to adjusting your habits to fit your current circumstances. The key is to maintain the core principles of healthy eating, regular physical activity, and self-care.

2. Fostering a Healthy Environment

Creating a Supportive Home Environment

Your home environment plays a significant role in supporting your new lifestyle. Make changes that encourage healthy habits and reduce temptations:

- **Stock Healthy Foods:** Keep your pantry and refrigerator filled with nutritious options and minimize junk food.
- **Organize Your Kitchen:** Make healthy cooking easier by organizing your kitchen and

keeping your cooking tools and ingredients accessible.

- **Create a Fitness Space:** Designate a space for exercise, whether it's a corner of your living room, a home gym, or a spot in your backyard.

Building a Supportive Social Network

Surround yourself with people who support your goals and encourage your healthy lifestyle. Communicate your needs and goals to friends and family, and seek their support. Join local or online communities that share your interests in health and wellness. Having a support network can provide motivation, accountability, and a sense of belonging.

Minimizing Environmental Triggers

Identify and minimize environmental triggers that may lead to unhealthy behaviors. For example:

- **Avoiding Temptations:** Keep tempting, unhealthy foods out of sight or out of the house altogether.
- **Limiting Screen Time:** Reduce sedentary behaviors by limiting time spent watching TV or using electronic devices.
- **Managing Stress:** Create a calm and organized living space to reduce stress and promote relaxation.

3. Spreading the Positive Influence

Sharing Your Journey

Sharing your weight loss journey can inspire and motivate others. Be open about your experiences, challenges, and successes. You can share your story through social media, blogs, or by talking with friends and family. Your journey can provide valuable insights and encouragement to those who are also working toward their health goals.

Becoming a Role Model

Lead by example and become a role model for healthy living. Your actions can influence others to make positive changes in their lives. Whether it's by demonstrating healthy eating habits, staying active, or managing stress effectively, your behavior can have a positive impact on those around you.

Supporting Others

Offer support and encouragement to others on their health journeys. This can be through:

- **Active Listening:** Provide a listening ear and understanding for friends and family who are working on their health goals.
- **Sharing Resources:** Share helpful resources such as recipes, workout routines, or wellness tips.
- **Creating Group Activities:** Organize group activities like healthy potlucks, fitness

challenges, or walking groups to foster a sense of community and mutual support.

4. Continuing Self-Improvement

Setting New Goals

After achieving your initial weight loss goals, it's important to set new goals to continue your journey of self-improvement. These goals can focus on various aspects of health and wellness, such as:

- **Fitness:** Training for a race, improving strength, or mastering a new sport.
- **Nutrition:** Trying new healthy recipes, experimenting with different diets (e.g., plant-based, Mediterranean), or focusing on micronutrient intake.
- **Mental Well-being:** Developing mindfulness practices, pursuing hobbies, or improving work-life balance.

Lifelong Learning

Commit to lifelong learning and staying informed about health and wellness. Read books, attend workshops, and follow credible sources of health information. The field of health and nutrition is constantly evolving, and staying informed can help you make the best choices for your well-being.

Embracing Change

Embrace change as a natural part of life and be open to evolving your habits and routines. Personal growth often involves stepping out of your comfort zone and trying new things. Whether it's a new exercise class, a different cooking technique, or a fresh perspective on self-care, be willing to experiment and adapt.

Practicing Self-Reflection

Regular self-reflection helps you stay connected to your goals and recognize areas for improvement. Take time to reflect on your progress, celebrate your achievements, and identify any challenges you need to address. Journaling can be an effective tool for self-reflection, allowing you to track your thoughts, feelings, and experiences over time.

Maintaining Balance

Strive for balance in all areas of your life. While maintaining a healthy lifestyle is important, it's equally important to enjoy life and find joy in your daily activities. Balance means allowing yourself to indulge occasionally, managing stress effectively, and nurturing your relationships. A balanced approach to health and wellness ensures that you can sustain your new lifestyle in the long term.

Embracing a new lifestyle is a continuous journey that requires commitment, flexibility, and a positive mindset. By making permanent changes, fostering a supportive environment, spreading positive influence, and continuing self-improvement, you can maintain your weight loss and enjoy a healthier, happier life. This final chapter underscores the importance of viewing weight loss not as a temporary goal but as a lifelong commitment to well-being and self-care.

AFTERWORD

The Journey Continues

Congratulations! By reaching the end of this book, you've taken a significant step toward transforming your life and achieving your weight loss goals. This journey is about more than just shedding pounds; it's about embracing a healthier, happier, and more fulfilling lifestyle.

Reflecting on Your Journey

Take a moment to reflect on the progress you've made. Consider the limiting beliefs you've challenged, the positive attitude you've cultivated, and the sustainable habits you've developed. Each chapter has provided you with tools and strategies to overcome obstacles and stay committed to your goals. Celebrate these accomplishments and recognize the hard work and dedication that has brought you to this point.

Embracing the Future

The path to a healthier life is ongoing. There will be ups and downs, but with the foundation you've built, you are well-equipped to handle them. Remember that setbacks are a natural part of any journey. When they occur, use the skills you've learned to stay resilient, motivated, and focused on your long-term vision.

Continue to set new goals, seek knowledge, and embrace change. Whether you're striving for further weight loss, improved fitness, or overall well-being, keep pushing yourself to grow and evolve. Stay curious, stay committed, and most importantly, stay kind to yourself.

Spreading the Positive Influence

Your journey doesn't end with you. By sharing your story and supporting others, you can contribute to a broader movement of health and wellness. Be a role model, offer encouragement, and create a ripple effect of positive change in your community. Your experiences and insights can inspire others to embark on their own journeys toward better health.

Final Thoughts

Weight loss for hopeless cases is not an impossible dream; it's a tangible goal that you can achieve with the right mindset, tools, and support. This book has aimed to empower you with knowledge and strategies to navigate your unique path to success. You have the power to transform your life, and every small step you take brings you closer to your ultimate goals.

Thank you for allowing this book to be part of your journey. May you continue to grow, thrive, and inspire those around you. Remember, the journey to health and happiness is not a destination but a lifelong adventure. Embrace it with open arms, and enjoy every step along the way.

To your health and happiness!

9 7 9 8 3 3 3 7 6 3 0 1 3